Intimate Invasions

the erotic ins & outs of enema play

by M.R. Strict

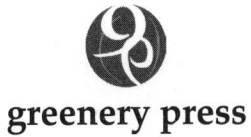

greenery press

Published in the United States by Greenery Press, 4200 Park Blvd. pmb 240, Oakland, CA 94602, *www.greenerypress.com*.

ISBN 1-890159-51-4.

CONTENTS

i. Author's Note i

ii. Prologue iii

Chapter 1: Initiation 1

Chapter 2: The Mechanics of Enema Administration 7

Chapter 3: The Enema Bandit 23

Chapter 4: A Phillipic on Morality 41

Chapter 5: The Reorientation 49

Chapter 6: The Punishment 61

Chapter 7: Twelve Steps to Effective Anticipation 73

Chapter 8: Over the Milking Stool 91

Chapter 9: Ageplay: from the "Punishment Book" 135

AUTHOR'S NOTE

Although this book is based my own extensive real-life experiences, some of the stories in it are obviously not real-life, but are instead fiction. Even so, these stories serve to enlarge the real-life applicability of the book by illustrating the erotic potential of the subject matter described herein. Invention may be one percent inspiration and 99 percent perspiration, but sex, done right, stands that proposition on its head. Specifically, the best sex is 99 percent inspirational, and only one percent perspirational – a proposition which should come as a relief both for those of us with bad backs and for all those readers dwelling in the desert southwest.

Three other points. First, all the real-world activities I describe in this book are consensual, as all such activities should be, including your own. Those fantasies that describe nonconsensual activity are intended as inspiration only, and as jumping-off points for your own fantasies and/or for fully consensual activities only.

Second, as a writer of a book for both men and women, I have struggled to keep my language as gender-neutral as possible while still keeping the book readable. Therefore, please recognize that sections of the book written to describe the interaction of a particular gender pair are transposable to any other pairwise combination of the sexes.

Finally, to my friends who helped review and edit this book, thank you. I could not have done this without your help.

PROLOGUE

I've based this book on the premise that the best kind of teaching is by graphic, visceral example, and not by step-by-step explication, not by the nuts-and-bolts approach. Therefore, although do I use nuts-and-bolts to explain the basics of how to give and receive an enema, for the most part I've focused on stories. The stories of people I've met and what I've done — or seen done — with them.

Enemas. I've given enemas, and seen them given, too many times to count. At home and on the road, in towns you'd be familiar with and in towns you've never heard of, tiny dots on detailed maps, little places that you'd barely notice even if you were driving right through them.

❋   ❋   ❋

Within these covers you'll find stories that encompass men and women in all possible combinations and of all orientations. Most of the stories are true; a few, which concern enemas given without the consent of the recipient, spring from my overheated imagination, and are not to be emulated except as a role-play between consenting and affectionate partners.

Why all these pairings? Because what I'm describing knows no boundaries of gender, knows no boundaries of dominance, or submission.

I hope you learn from what you read, from each interaction, from all of them. And I hope you'll learn from the nuts-and-bolts sections in this book that help fill in the details. Dominance and submission pervade human interactions, and the more you understand that, the more you understand humans. And yourself, your own interests in the topic. I've spent some fifteen years trying to understand the emotions that underpin the acts. I hope I convey some of what I've learned to you.

* * *

So, come now. Escape. Step into your car, close the door and drive, down the pavement and out of the town where you live, out of the safety of your usual frame of reference and into the *terra incognita* of *my* world, a world without preconception.

A world of endless potentials: a woman here, a man there. A couple, waiting outside the hotel door. Or inside their bedroom.

Pack lightly: all you'll need is the desire to leave the world you live in now.

Which is more easily arranged than you might think.

INITIATION

She lies over his lap, feeling his fingers in the waistband of her panties. All too aware that, once he has pulled them down, she is going to receive the first enema of her life.

She knows she presents a tantalizing view, her crack visible to him through the transparent seat of her underpants, her behind framed by her raised skirt above, the garter straps to either side, the black stockings below.

She groans with humiliation, knowing how much of her is on display, knowing that, despite her dread of the enema, she is aroused, and that her arousal is apparent to him. He's commented on it, put his fingers between her legs and pushed into her sodden sex through the fabric of the underpants, told her how naughty she is.

He's told her that he intends to masturbate her while she gets the enema, a fact that terrifies her even more than the enema itself, for she doesn't know if she can retain during orgasm. She pleads with him, but his resolve is apparent. He tells her that naughty girls get punished, and that her punishment is to come while the soapy water rushes into her virgin bowels. To come while bent over his lap, panties down to her knees, the thick nozzle pushed up her Vaselined anus, squirming and shifting as the water rushes into her bowels and his hand tickles her between her legs.

To come while she is getting her first enema, over his lap crying and squirming to retain while he describes to her how much he enjoys the sight her bared bottom presents with the nozzle inserted into it.

To come while he tells her that the enema is only the first, and that she's going to get her bottom thoroughly cleaned before he enters her there, fucks her ass hard for the first time in her life.

She is understandably nervous at this thought.

And she is also very very wet.

* * *

The panties are coming down now, and she feels their descent. He is unhurried in his motions, toying with the thin fabric, toying with her as well. She knows this, resents it. But at the same time she is aware that it's all part of the process, a rainbow arc, a rocket's trajectory that starts at the ground, climbs slowly up through the stratosphere, and, finally, reaches the zenith of orgasm.

He has emphasized the importance of ritual. Has told her that each step leads inevitably to the next, and that the progression is important, will help her locate herself in the process, help her prepare herself mentally for what's coming.

He's told her that it's a natural human need, this ritual. He's emphasized the childish aspects of what he does, emphasized the loss of control he's going to make sure she experiences. The sense of regression, of being small, cared for, looked after... all thoughts she'll feel that will comfort her as he bares her behind, spreads her cheeks, puts the nozzle in, opens the clamp. And rubs between her legs as she squirms and shifts over his lap, feeling the pressure in her bowels grow.

* * *

She feels him pulling her panties down, feels the slow descent, the gradual baring of her behind to the cold air and, worse, his gaze. She feels childish, having her bottom exposed, feels like crying out, pleading with him, "daddy, please..." but keeps quiet, realizing how much more humiliating it will be when she breaks down and begs.

She lies there, feeling the solidity of his legs under her, feels the lump in the center of his lap that she knows marks his own excitement at what he's having to do. Somehow this excitement of his is comforting, makes her feel loved. It also increases her own arousal, to know how much he's enjoying the baring of her behind, how excited he is to be in control of her, of her little rear hole and what has to go in it. Soon.

She bends over his lap feeling her panties come down, listening to him scold. Her focus is imperfect; at times she is able to concentrate on his words, but often she drifts off into a mental fog, where all she can do is feel, where speech is beyond her capacity. He is all too aware of her mental state, it seems, for every time she begins to lose herself he punctuates his scolding with a sharp smack to her behind, the impact shaking her back into the reality of her situation.

She imagines that reality for a moment. Bare-bottomed, panties halfway down her thighs, behind stuck up, legs too far apart for comfort. She imagines someone looking in the window and seeing her this way, a naughty girl, about to be taught a lesson.

He is hard, she is wet... and the nozzle is something she can already feel entering her, forcing its way up her virgin behind. Lodging itself deep in her bowels, the discomfort as palpable as the excitement she expects it to bring. She can already feel it there, deep in her posterior, intruding, and teasing. She can feel it, even though in fact it's still on the table by her head.

She is almost inclined to look at it, to see its thickness, and the thick coating of Vaseline he's applied to it. Instead, she puts her head down and focuses on the descent of her panties, and the sight her bare bottom presents to him.

She feels his cock grow even harder underneath her.

❅ ❅ ❅

He leans forward to the table beside them and retrieves something. Bent over, head down towards the floor, she is unable to see what it is that he's picked up, but she knows from what she's seen on the table that it can only mean more embarrassment for her.

This conclusion is confirmed when she hears the sound of a package being opened, and then the snap of a rubber glove. He's told her he's going to do an examination first; in fact, this was one of the things he emphasized when they first talked, when she asked him why he would give her an enema, how he would know she had to have one.

"I'll do an examination, of course," he replied, so matter-of-factly that it took a moment for his words to sink in. "An examination..." she repeated, aware suddenly of her burning face, "an... examination...?"

"Yes, of your behind, the state of your behind," he replied, "with a gloved finger while you behave yourself and keep still." She hesitated, asked him what he meant, but the phone in her hand was silent for a long time before he replied. And, when he finally did answer, it was to tell her that it was something she would just have to find out for herself when the time came.

The conversation was distressing, she recalls; more distressing still was the fact that she ran through it time and time again in her mind as she lay in bed in the weeks that followed. Imagining him undressing her, or at least her bottom, baring her so that she was ready for it. Perhaps he had a stool or table she would have to bend over to have her panties pulled down, as they did it in the doctor's office. Or would he take the more juvenile approach and put her over his knees? Or – the worst she could imagine – would he have her get on the bed or a low table with her behind up and her head down? She's ashamed to admit she actually tried this position a few times, reached back and pulled her panties down, imagining it was his hand doing it. And then knelt there feeling how opened her rear cheeks were, knowing he would be able to see between them, see the tightened little hole, waiting to be penetrated, so small, so vulnerable.

And now, it's not just her imagination. The snap of the glove behind her is real, and she feels the cold feeling of his gloved fingers going between her cheeks, spreading them.

She knows what he sees: her virginal bottomhole, tensing, waiting for its first penetration.

And, his finger teasing that bottomhole, just the Vaselined tip intruding, pushing slightly, just enough to cause her to moan slightly.

She knows that moan gets louder as the finger pushes in firmly, disappears inside her tight behind.

She shifts over his lap, for some odd reason coming to rest with his knee more firmly between her legs.

He chooses to ignore her presumptiveness. The finger goes deeper.

And the moan? It gets louder still.

* * *

He's scolding again, moving his finger in and out as he chides her for her behavior, picking one embarrassing topic after another for his lecture.

He's right in what he says, each point he makes is a fair one. Much worse, however, he drives his finger home into her bottom to emphasize each statement, his voice rising and falling, his finger moving in and out in synchrony. She is red-faced, and recognizes those familiar feelings between her legs that demonstrate that blood is flowing to other parts of her as well. She feels humiliated to be over his knees like this, panties down... but the arousal offsets the humiliation, and she finds herself pushing up off his lap to get more of his finger inside her each time he withdraws it. She realizes she's sodomizing herself on it, realizes the humiliation of that act. Once again, the humiliation, instead of quenching her arousal, inflames it.

On and on he lectures, and she knows he sees her moving, feels her rise and fall over his knees. She also knows he feels her behind tighten on him each time he pushes his finger in, knows he smells her arousal. She should be ashamed – and she is, really – but that shame only feeds her desire, only pushes her on to even greater acts of depravity.

On and on he lectures, letting his finger move freely in her behind as he does. She feels him begin to move it from side to side slightly, and she knows he's inspecting her, assaying her cleanliness. With this knowledge an even greater mortification overcomes her.

In and out his finger moves, and she knows he's checking, trying to determine how many enemas he's going to give her. It's her first time, she's never had one before, and she's pleaded with him to limit the treatment to a single bagful. But he's refused to negotiate; instead, he's told her that it will be up to him. The whole topic has caused her enormous anxiety; still, she trusts him, knows he is careful. And, deep down, understands that it's all part of that process of letting go, of giving up control to him. However many he ultimately decides she needs to have.

In and out, in and out. Finally, he stops, holds it in, all the way up her behind.

He says nothing. Just keeps her there, impaled on his finger.

He says nothing; even so, she knows it's time.

This knowledge is confirmed when he withdraws his finger, lifts her off his lap and leads her to the corner. Has her wait there, bare bottom on display, nose to the wall, as he walks out of the room.

She hears him in the bathroom. Hears the water running in the sink.

And knows that, when he returns, he will be holding the enema bag.

She wonders how big the nozzle will be.

And how it will feel sliding up her behind.

THE MECHANICS OF ENEMA ADMINISTRATION

---

1.   The Basic Kinds of Enemas: Solutions

An enema works to stimulate the bowels, of course, but that stimulation can take one of several forms. It can be the result of a simple volume effect, where the amount of solution causes the need. Or, it can be the consequence of the nature of the solution administered: some solutions cause an increase in water volume in the intestines; others act to mildly irritate the intestines and thereby produce an effect.

Here I'm going to talk about two premixed solutions, chemical, and oil, both packaged into enemas by the Fleet company, as well as under more generic brand names. I'm also going to discuss the basic solutions that can be mixed at home: salty water, and the soapsuds enema (SSE).

And after that, I'm going to conclude this section with a brief discussion of other solutions, basically to point out that, although people do use them, I don't, and can't recommend their use to others. Without further ado:

- **The Fleet™ Chemical Enema.** If there's one type of enema that people encounter most regularly, it's this one, also known generically as a Fleet enema. An enema given in the hospital is usually a Fleet, for the simple reason that this kind of enema is small, easy to administer, and produces results quickly. For exactly these reasons, the first enema you might find yourself giving — or receiving — will probably be a Fleet.

    That said, what are the ins and outs of a Fleet enema? Well, a Fleet isn't much to look at, a not especially sexy small plastic squeeze-bottle with a flexible tip that serves as the nozzle. Remove the cap that covers the pre-lubricated tip, insert the tip into the appropriate backside, and squeeze the bottle. That's it as far as complexity goes, at least for administration. The only thing that need be said, in passing, is that the Fleet is most conveniently administered over-the-knee, a particularly juvenile position about which I shall be saying more presently.

Once the solution goes in, things get more interesting. As noted above, a Fleet is a class of enema that I loosely term a chemical enema. A Fleet works by drawing water into the bowels; the larger volume of water creates the urge to go. The question is, how strong is that need, and how does it compare to the need created by the other types of enemas? I leave a longer discussion on the sensations themselves to a separate section below.

In my experience the effects of a Fleet vary widely: for some, the sensation is slight and their ability to retain great; for others, the sensation is large and, not surprisingly, the ability to retain very poor. I've never understood why this should be, but it is. There is no doubt that, like any other kind of enema, administration of a Fleet shortly after a meal is more problematic than administration several hours after eating, when retention is much easier; the more specific effects of a Fleet on any particular individual otherwise require an empirical approach. That is, try one and see what the reaction is.

Now, before closing out this section, I want to talk briefly about the *chemical* nature of Fleet enemas. People are afraid of chemicals, especially chemicals injected into such an intimate part of the body. So the obvious question is, what are the effects of taking a Fleet? Are there dangerous chemicals in them that are harmful?

Answer: emphatically *no*, with a few provisos. I suppose the most obvious facts — that Fleet enemas are commonly used by hospitals and are available without prescription at any drugstore — should be evidence enough that Fleet enemas are safe. But let me reiterate: Fleet enemas are safe, as long as you obey a few simple rules about using them.

First, Fleets, like any enemas, should not be used regularly, although "regularity" is somewhat subject to interpretation. Basically, tampering with the normal course of excretion is a bad idea, and the body will become dependent on enemas for bowel activity if they're used too frequently. Daily use is too frequent. Once a month isn't. Once a week? I don't know that there is any simple answer, but I would advise against this high a frequency of use, at least as a matter of course.

Second, Fleets — again like any enemas — should not be used where there are medical problems in the recipient. These include the obvious, like perforations in the bowel, etc. But they should also not be used when the patient has heart or renal (kidney) disease, at least not without consulting a doctor. (See p. 16 for more information on medical considerations.)

Again, though, I want to emphasize that, used correctly by people in good health, enemas are completely safe.

- **The Oil Enema.** I include oil enemas mostly for completeness, for this category of enema really doesn't induce expulsion as much as it does facilitate it; there is a volume of oil introduced which may stimulate the need, but mostly the oil acts to soften the material inside and thereby facilitate its expulsion.

Oil enemas do still have their place in the pantheon of punishment, for the simple reason that, like the other enemas discussed, they are intrusive, and they are *preparatory*, a psychological factor that is always powerful, no matter what end goal the person administering the enema has in mind.

Oil enemas are sold in the same squeeze bottles that hold Fleet chemical enemas, and administration of an oil enema is consequently identical to administration of a chemical enema. Retention and expulsion of an oil enema are, however, not at all similar.

Retention of an oil enema is not difficult: there is no great tendency to expel the oil. On the other hand, there is a high chance of oil leaking out of its own accord, and that makes oil enemas inherently messier. If you give an oil enema, make sure that there is a pad of some kind between the recipient's posterior and clothing, bed, or what have you; if there isn't, you are guaranteed an oil spot.

Expulsion of an oil enema is also problematic, in that there is always residual oil left afterwards. The only sure way of completely removing the oil is to follow expulsion with one or more water enemas, a fact that should always be kept in mind when you are planning to give (or take) an oil enema.

- **The Salt-Water Enema.** Unlike a chemical enema, a saltwater enema consists quite simply of water and salt, about one tablespoon per two quarts. The salt acts to maintain the electrolyte balance; that is, to help prevent the loss of salts from the body into the water injected into the bowels.

  A salt-water enema is generally larger than a chemical enema, although it doesn't have to be. In terms of intended, medicinal purpose — bowel cleansing — an enema of this type is usually larger because it doesn't contain chemicals to induce a large volume in the intestine nor irritant soap to stimulate the bowels to action. But remember, we aren't generally talking intended purpose here — we're talking psychological and physical effects, embarrassment and the intrusiveness of the whole process. Therefore the volume used in a salt-water enema can be anything from a few drops up to the reasonable maximum of two quarts (for experienced recipients).

  That said, pretty clearly the ability to retain is dependent mostly upon the amount of solution administered. Give a small volume and retention will be fairly easy. Give a larger volume and retention becomes harder. Psychodrama is heightened with larger volumes, although giving a small volume with longer retention while a larger volume is prepared in front of the culprit can have an effect every bit as great as having the culprit watch as a full bag is prepared for immediate administration.

- **The Soapsuds Enema (SSE).** A soapsuds enema (SSE) works by a combination of solution volume and mild irritation by the soap in the solution. Emphasis there on *mild* irritation — do *not* use a harsh soap, only a mild white hand soap such as Ivory™, which can be dissolved in the water beforehand until the solution is milky white.

Like a saltwater enema, a SSE is more or less difficult to retain depending upon the volume administered. A SSE is certainly harder to hold than one of plain water, and usually harder than a Fleet. I suppose it's fair to say that the SSE is the most threatening of the enemas I'm going to describe, because of the actual effects of the solution, because of the threatening nature of the soapy water itself, and because, like a saltwater enema, SSEs are often given using an enema bag, which is threatening.

- **Other Solutions.** There are many other solutions that can be used in enemas apart from the ones I've described above. I'm not going to talk about these variants, for one simple reason: *safety*. The solutions I've described are mild enough and commonly enough used in hospitals and by medical professionals, that it's pretty clear that with minor precautions they can be used without danger by those not formally trained. But this is not the case with many of the other solutions people sometimes describe, and for that reason I can't recommend them.

  Now this is not to say that these other solutions are necessarily unsafe; and I'm sure there will be some people reading who will scoff at my cautiousness. My answer is simple, though: so much of the effect of an enema is either emotional or can be elicited through straightforward solutions that I don't see the need to discuss other concoctions, even if I thought that they were safe enough to suggest to everyone.

  And some concoctions are quite dangerous. Thus my admonishment to stick with what I've described, premixed Fleet chemical enemas, oil enemas, and salt and soapsuds enemas.

---

2.   *The Basic Kinds of Enemas: Equipment*

The basic purpose of an enema is to produce the need to expel. That is accomplished by the solution injected and, as I have discussed above, there are really a fairly limited number of solutions you should use to achieve this effect.

On the other hand, the *ways* of administering enemas are quite a bit more varied, and exciting. I'm reminded of the Rime of the Ancient Mariner, "He … loveth best all things, both great and small." As you shall see, apparatus for the administration of enemas falls quite nicely into those two categories.

- **Small Things: The Rectal Syringe.** I use "Rectal Syringe" to describe both Fleet chemical and oil enemas, and to describe enemas given with what in drugstores are actually sold as rectal syringes: a rubber squeeze bulb with a hard plastic nozzle about 2 1/2 inches long and perhaps 1/4 inch in diameter attached at one end.

  The attraction of the rectal syringe, in any of these forms, is that it's just the right size and shape to be used over the knee, a particularly embarrassing and juvenile position. In hospitals a Fleet is given with the patient on the left side, right leg drawn up to the chest, for reasons having to do with efficacy of penetration of the solution into the turns of the bowels. In general, though, I much prefer over the knee, so that the culprit can look down at the floor and feel his or her cheeks being separated, knowing I'm enjoying the view, seeing those bare cheeks and the little hole between them.

  The second attraction of the rectal syringe, in the case where it's to be used to administer a salt-water or soapy water enema, is that it has to be refilled and reinserted and squeezed quite a few times to administer the same volume as a bag enema. And each of those steps has a particular poignancy and power: the first filling, usually done from a basin of water by the culprit's head, the culprit watching out of the corner of his or her eye as the bulb is squeezed and the tip is submerged in the water, the sound of the water being sucked into the bulb, and then the tickling insertion; and then of course once the thin lubricated nozzle is deep in the "patient's" behind, the second squeeze, this time to administer the solution, a process that can be as slow or as fast, as gentle or as vigorous as the person giving the enema desires.

The third attraction of the rectal syringe is that it is particularly convenient to carry — more than once I've taken a Fleet with me to parties and, when my companion has misbehaved, taken her panties down in a back bedroom and put her over my lap for the rapid — and relentless — administration of liquid justice. Even when I give a water or soapsuds enema I often use a rectal syringe for its convenience: no bag to fill, no hook to find to hang it from. Just the syringe, the basin of water and the culprit, bare red bottom over my lap.

To recap then, the rectal syringe — Fleet or actual rectal syringe as sold in a drugstore — is: convenient to use; particularly sensation-provoking because, for the administration of larger volumes, it has to be reinserted a number of times; and, particularly suited to juvenile regression, because it is conveniently given over the lap, a very childish posture to be in.

• **"Great" Things: The Bag Enema.** There's no doubt that the bag enema is intimidating: the bulging reservoir, dangling hose and thick nozzle cannot fail to immediately conjure images of penetration and loss of control. That said, it's important to remember that both the bag enema and the rectal syringe can be used to great effect, and that under some circumstances the threat of the rectal syringe is every bit as unnerving as the threat of the full bag.

The threat of the full bag. Let's talk about that for a moment. As mentioned, a bag enema consists of a fluid reservoir, usually rubber, usually red if you've purchased the most common kind of bag enema, a combination hot water bottle/douche/ enema bag; a hose which connects to the bag and, at the other end, to the nozzle; and the nozzle itself, which can range from the small white plastic nozzle packaged with a combo bag to something far more esoteric, a double-Bardex nozzle for example (see p. 14). The threat comes from the size of the bag and from the nozzle that the disciplinarian has attached to the end of the hose.

Although the reservoir of a bag enema contains roughly two quarts of water (more for some hospital bags and for high volume bags that some specialty vendors provide), there is no particular reason why the reservoir needs to be completely filled. On the other hand, a fully filled bag has the maximum psychological effect on the recipient: even if he or she isn't going to end up getting all of it, knowing that the disciplinarian can choose to administer the full two quart load is daunting, and adds to both the corrective process and the loss of control the recipient needs to feel during the administration and retention.

Adding to the psychological effect of the bag enema is the nozzle. A combination hot water bottle/douche bag/enema bag includes two nozzles: a small enema nozzle and a larger douche nozzle. Either can be used to administer an enema; the douche nozzle used for this purpose imparts both greater stimulation and a greater degree of intimidation as well. There are other nozzles that can be used, a topic I'll cover in the next section.

Finally, a bag enema is unique in that the large volume of water in the reservoir can be administered slowly, quickly, or in-between, with frequent clamping off of the hose while the culprit is chided for his or her behavior. A scolding that the penitent usually has trouble hearing because he or she is too worried about hearing the loud *click* that signals the resumption of the flow of solution into the naughty backside.

Oh, and one other thing. You can spank the culprit during the administration of a bag enema. Not over the nozzle, of course, but to either side. A rich mélange of sensations. No doubt you will want to try it, whether you're administering the enema and spanking, or receiving them.

- **The Bardex and Double-Bardex Nozzles.** There are three things you need to know about Bardex nozzles: they're expensive; they're high-maintenance; and, they're worth having!

Bardex nozzles are basically nozzles that have one (single-Bardex) or two (double-Bardex) balloons on the end. In a single-Bardex there is one balloon, which can be inflated inside the recipient's behind once the balloon is inserted (deflated the balloon is relatively easy to get in). In a double-Bardex there are two balloons, one that's inflated inside the bottom in question, another that's inflated outside. The idea behind the double-Bardex is that the two balloons squeeze the bottom-hole between them, ensuring that nothing leaks out until the balloons are deflated and removed. The same thing goes for the single-Bardex, of course, just not quite to the same extent.

Bardexes, single or double, are usually made of latex rubber, although less expensive versions can be obtained where a thin rubber balloon is attached to the exterior of a hard plastic nozzle. Latex Bardexes are superior, in longevity and certainly in appearance, but latex Bardexes are also quite expensive. Expect to spend at least $70 on a single-Bardex and well over $100 for a double-Bardex made of latex.

A latex Bardex requires particular care in its use. First, the balloons should not be over-inflated, or they will pop (and even if they don't pop, over-inflation is bad for the behind of the person the inner balloon is being inflated in). The general rule is two squeezes of the rubber inflation bulb that either accompanies the Bardex or that you've bought to accompany it. Second, only use a water-soluble lubricant on a Bardex; that means KY jelly or something like it, and not Vaseline. If you use Vaseline you'll destroy the Bardex, since Vaseline rots the rubber (and, incidentally, will do the same to the rubber in condoms — something to keep in mind if you want to practice safe sex afterwards, when the last residues of Vaseline are still there despite your best efforts at removing them). And, third, be fastidious about cleaning the Bardex (warm soapy water and then plain water rinse), drying it thoroughly, and storing it out of the sun.

All that said, the Bardex nozzles are incredible to use or receive because they prevent expulsion, and in fact were developed for medical use in procedures requiring long retentions. Now infinitely long retention isn't a good idea, but having a nozzle that can be used in a balky bottom, or with a recalcitrant recipient to ensure they hold the solution for as long as needed — that's a nozzle you can't do without. Also, there's the little matter of how the nozzle feels inflated in the behind of the culprit; not to mention how it looks, especially if it's a double-Bardex and you can see the exterior balloon inflated between the penitent's cheeks.

One last thing. Let's say you've bought a double-Bardex and have used it on one person and now have someone new you want to use it with. Bite the bullet and don't use it. It isn't sanitary to use any enema equipment with a second person, especially not a nozzle that can't be sterilized. It may hurt to contemplate having to spend $100 or more to buy a second Bardex for your new love, but it's completely irresponsible to use the Bardex you've used before with someone else.

And by the same token, if you're the recipient, at the very least ask if the nozzle is new. Ideally, bring your own equipment; it may not be as sexy, but it's safe. And that's no little issue to ignore.

---

3.   *Enema Safety*

As I've already discussed, enemas are basically quite safe. They are used regularly in hospitals, and are available without prescription at any drugstore. That said there are some basic precautions you need to follow when administering/receiving enemas, precautions I've laid out below.

• **Medical Issues.** There are two basic issues to be considered, health-wise, as you think about indulging in this most erotic of pastimes. Neither should preclude you from enjoying enemas (unless your intended recipient suffers from heart disease, kidney disorders, or bowel problems — in which case he or she *must* consult a physician, who does not need to know that the enemas aren't for constipation).

   First, the wall of the bowel is not really a "wall," it's more of a sponge. Any substance that flows into the bowel is rapidly soaked up by the blood vessels there, and thus into the body's other systems.

Occasionally, in the wrong kind of pornographic literature, you'll read about enemas containing alcoholic beverages. Any such inclusion bypasses the body's normal systems for processing alcohol and is quite dangerous, and is vigorously not recommended here.

More to the point, the fluid of which our bodies are made is, as we all learned in grade school, salt water, of the approximate salinity of the ocean. Thus, if we use plain water in our enema bags, our bodies will eagerly soak up the plain water across the bowel wall, and we will find ourselves peeing vastly for several hours after our enema adventures. This is not generally a problem, but if you wish to prevent it (if, for example, you would like to have a good long sleep afterwards), simply add some salt to your enema solution, one teaspoon of table salt to one quart of water.

Second, anal penetration, in most people, causes a neurological reflex which causes (in varying degrees) some slowing of the heartbeat, along with a general feeling of languor. Some people may feel tearful, lightheaded, shaky or physically weak. Fainting ("syncope" is the medical term) is an unusual but not unheard-of outcome.

Given that many people interpret these feelings as feelings of sensuality or submissiveness, they are generally a positive outcome in our world — but, for the enema recipient with health problems, they can be genuinely worrisome or even dangerous; and for the couple not expecting them, they can be startling. For the enema recipient in good health, they are generally nothing to worry about. However, it's a good idea to position such a person in such a way that if they become light-headed, a fall will not harm them.

If fainting seems imminent, remove any foreign objects from the rectum and place the individual on the toilet, head between knees, to expel. If fainting actually takes place, place the individual on her back (I'll assume, for pronoun ease, that the recipient is a female) and check pulse and breathing. She should come around within a minute or two.

If she has no pulse or is not breathing, call 911 immediately — the situation has become a serious medical emergency. This outcome is wildly unlikely, and I have no wish to be a killjoy, but since the possibility — albeit slight — is real, it needs to be discussed. In the same vein, I strongly recommend that you obtain and maintain a current first aid/CPR card, whether or not you ever give or receive another enema — it's just a good idea.

- **New Equipment (Sharing Is Not Always A Good Thing).** Enema equipment used on someone new should always be new; sharing equipment that's been used with someone else is unsafe, even if it's been thoroughly cleaned and disinfected. There's really no excuse for not using new equipment anyway; apart from Bardex nozzles and some other types of expensive equipment, most enema apparatus is either disposable or very inexpensive.

  Enema equipment used with the same person should be left with that person; in fact, ideally the person receiving the enema should provide the equipment, on the theory that if its going in your behind then you ought to know exactly where it came from. Routinely used equipment can be kept sanitary with soap and water; after washing, rubber items should be dried as thoroughly as possible in order to prevent them from discoloring, and should be stored out of the sun, which also destroys rubber.

  Let me repeat, equipment should never be shared. And in case you're wondering, this maxim applies to fluid reservoirs and tubing, not just to nozzles. While water seeks the lowest level, administered fluids have a way of working their way back up hoses into enema bags, and it's just plain not worth taking chances.

- **Solution Temperature and Pressure.** Hot water should never be used for an enema — if water is too hot to bathe in, it's far too hot for an enema. Lukewarm is the best temperature, but slightly cold water can also be used, although there will be considerably more cramping with colder water.

  As far as pressure goes, it can't be much of a surprise that fluids injected up the bottom shouldn't be given at high pressure; blow air into one end of a sausage — blow it hard — and the sausage bursts. It's exactly the same with the bowels, and that sort of scenario is just not one you want to explore.

Happily, pressure isn't a concern as long as you never ever use enemas that connect directly to the faucet or hang the fluid reservoir more than about 2 1/2 feet above the nozzle.

With regard to direct faucet attachment, a number of manufacturers sell hoses that have a nozzle at one end and an adapter at the other that allows you to connect up to a faucet. Bad idea. Sudden surges in water pressure can generate high pressures, and those pressures can be incredibly dangerous. Simple rule: never connect up to the faucet. It's much too dangerous.

With regard to bag heieght, if you hang an enema bag from the ceiling and put the recipient on the floor it may look exciting, it may be exciting to open the clamp and see the recipient's distress at the sudden influx of fluid, but it isn't safe. Fluid pressure builds the higher the reservoir is above the nozzle. The safe distance is a maximum of about 2 1/2 feet. Lower means slower flow, which is useful with someone who has problems retaining. Higher? Not safe. Don't try it. There's plenty of variety that you can obtain without exploring that particular aspect of enemas.

- **Nozzle Insertion.** Some nozzles are designed for deep insertion; strictly speaking they aren't nozzles at all, they're colon tubes or rectal tubes. Deep insertion carries with it the danger of rupturing the bowel wall with the end of the tube. In general you shouldn't put things in more than two inches. Leave deep insertion to the experts. Again, there's plenty to experiment with already.

- **Retention.** Generally, retention lasts anywhere from 5 seconds (grounds for spanking) to twenty minutes or so (grounds for compliments). I've heard stories about people made to retain for hours, and that's not a particularly great idea, unless it's an oil enema that's been given. The half-hour-or-less window is plenty for almost any scenario.

- **Frequency of Administration.** As previously discussed, enemas should not be given too frequently: less than once a week. High frequency results in a dependency on enemas for bowel movements and can also alter the intestinal flora for the worse.

- **Multiple Enemas.** A single enema does not completely clean out the recipient's behind; in order to accomplish that goal, at least two or three enemas are required. Multiple enemas are not dangerous, as long as the procedure isn't repeated every night, but multiple enemas are rather tiring for the recipient, and may cause a certain amount of dehydration. Drinking orange juice helps, but this is not the only precaution one should take.

  Multiple enemas are obviously the best preparation for other anal activities, such as the penetration of the culprit's behind with a plug, a strap-on, or something fleshier. However, be advised that multiple enemas do cause a certain amount of soreness, something that needs to be considered, especially if the person receiving them is inexperienced in that area.

  Finally, multiple enemas should not be given to someone who has never had any enemas; intensity is exciting, but should be approached cautiously. Or to put it a little differently, "the best things come to those that wait."

---

4. *Positioning*

In hospitals, enemas are usually given with the patient on the left side, right leg drawn up to the chest. This position is favored because the colon turns in such a way that an enema given on the left side penetrates more deeply into the bowels.

Given that the enemas discussed in this book are *decidedly* non-medicinal, there is no particular reason to use this position; I prefer over-the-knee (OTK), face down on the bed, kneeling with head down, or even over the rim of a bathtub. A standing position is the one position that I don't really recommend, for the simple reason that gravity forces the fluid down, making the administration of any reasonable volume difficult.

On the other hand, a standing position is fine once the solution has gone in; it's harder to retain standing, so corner time while holding in the solution becomes that much more of a challenge

---

5.   *Administration*

There is no particular rule for administering enemas; the solution can be administered quickly or slowly depending upon the circumstances. Of course rapid administration is likely to cause more problems with retention, but again, that's a decision made on the basis of the circumstances rather than on any theoretical grounds.

The most important thing in administering an enema is to make sure that there is communication between the disciplinarian and the penitent; the sensations are very physical, and if the recipient says that he or she can't hold the solution, or that there are cramps, it's the responsibility of the person giving the enema to pay attention to those statements. To some extent they can be ignored — if it's a punishment enema it should be at least a little uncomfortable. But, as mentioned, the sensations are very real and cannot be denied. Pay attention to them.

---

6.   *Retention*

Retention and expulsion are two topics that are usually the most difficult to talk about. Why? Utter embarrassment, mostly from the thought of not being able to keep the fluid inside, and what that is like when it comes out.

Now, retention can be made easier or harder by varying the type of solution administered, how much is given, and of course how long it has to be retained. As I mentioned previously, apart from oil enemas, retention should generally be limited to a half hour or less. Whether or not the person retaining can actually make it to a half hour is a different story. Kindness dictates that you start with a short retention period and work your way up; start with too long a retention and the culprit won't be able to retain, leading to a scene that, given the intensity of enema play in general, may be more than either party wants.

Apart from solution temperature (lukewarm), volume (small), and speed of administration (slow), enema retention can also be encouraged by the use of a rectal plug after administration or by a single- or double-Bardex nozzle. Although it's not the optimum position for retaining an enema, I usually follow the administration of the fluid with time spent in the corner with the culprit bare-bottomed. The feeling of a red behind exposed, and the fullness in the tummy is, I'm told, quite profound. The piquancy of the situation can be increased by leaving the nozzle and dangling hose in the recipient's behind during corner time (assuming you've given a bag enema); having to walk to the corner and then stand there with the hose hanging down like a tail is very embarrassing. Which, of course, is exactly the point.

---

7.   *Expulsion*

Probably the most embarrassing aspect of enemas. I have a simple theory about expulsion: expulsion of the first enema should always be allowed in private. After that, privacy is up to the disciplinarian.

That said, keep in mind that of all the issues surrounding enemas, this is the one that will be the biggest bone of contention. For the recipient, having to expel will be embarrassing even in private; having to expel in front of the disciplinarian is so emotionally charged an experience that it should not be undertaken until a real rapport exists between the two parties. I am not in the least against requiring expulsion in front of me; but I don't require that until I have established what the comfort zone of the recipient is, and set up a situation in which pushing the very limit of that zone will lead to an intense but not destructive experience.

THE ENEMA BANDIT

The infamous ski bandit, who terrorized citizens by breaking into homes and giving enemas to females, may be operating again. The police reported five different incidents of a man breaking into two apartments and administering enemas to five different girls in the early morning hours, Friday.

The first incident happened at 2:54 a.m. There are three girls living in the apartment. Two of them were given enemas.

The second incident happened at 3:30 a.m. at another apartment complex, where the masked intruder walked in and gave three girls enemas.

Police said the intruder walked through doors — which the residents had left unlocked — tied the girls up after asking them to strip, talked gently to them, took their temperature and gave them enemas with a hot water bottle.

The police reported all the girls were students. At the first apartment all three girls were preparing to take a roommate, who complained of being sick, to the hospital.

As they walked out of their bedroom, they saw the man in the middle of their living room. The girls described the man as wearing a pillow case over his head with eye holes cut out.

After giving the enemas to two of the girls, sparing the girl who was going to the hospital, he cut the telephone line in the apartment and said not to call the police for five minutes.

At the second apartment two of the four occupants were studying when they heard someone walking in the front room of their apartment.

Moments later a man, with a pillowcase over his head, walked in. The intruder had the girls wake up the two who were sleeping. He told them what he was going to do and told them to relax, that "he had done it before," police were told.

✳ ✳ ✳

I think I'm most struck by the bathtub: large, one of those sauna-tubs, with water jets in the sides, a tub for luxuriating, not the usual utilitarian catch-basin for shower runoff.

A tub this big offers up possibilities all its own, and I study it carefully, sitting on the side looking down into it, imagining her kneeling there, head down, rump high. In that position the cheeks spread apart, and I imagine her looking at me pleadingly as I take her into the bathroom and stand her in the tub, telling her what I'm about to do as I fill and hang the bag from the towel rack.

The curtain is pulled back as she stands there watching me hang the bag, and she blanches when I calmly tell her it's time for her to have her pants down. I have her face the wall and I take a long minute to study her backside through the thin material of her pajama bottoms. The cheeks clench and loosen, and I enjoy looking at their heavy round fullness.

I put my hand out, flatten it on the surface of her backside, rub it up and down as I talk to her. I'm telling her to be calm, that I won't hurt her, and all the while I'm letting her feel my hand rubbing up and down her rump, letting her know without saying it how much it turns me on, focusing all her attention on what's behind her. In my mind she's letting her head hang down, but I can see a little bit of her face as I smooth my hand over her bum and tell her what I'm going to have to do. I watch her expression as I calmly describe the procedure, how in a minute I'm going to have to take her pajama bottoms down to her knees and then have her kneel down in the tub with her head down on its surface and her bottom up high. I pause my hand as I talk to her, and begin to push my finger gently into the crack between her cheeks as I talk, letting her feel it intruding slightly there. I tell her that, when she's kneeling, her cheeks will spread of their own accord for me, and that I'll have her wait there patiently as I prepare the nozzle. I imagine holding up the nozzle, showing it to her before I have her kneel, showing her the nozzle, and the jar of Vaseline. I continue to tickle between her cheeks with my finger as I hold up the nozzle close to her face and let her look at how thick it is, how long it is. Let her look at it. Let her think about where it's going.

I stand up and look down into the tub, and imagine her standing there. I have both hands in the waistband of her pajamas now, fingertips pressing lightly into her warm flesh, having her face the wall as I tell her that it's time for her pants to come down. And the do come down, slowly; I watch as they come down exposing the bottom curve of her back, and then the top of her bottom. I pull a little more and both cheeks come into view, two round cheeks with the hidden valley in between. I pull the bottoms down slowly, letting her feel more and more exposed as the fabric descends, letting her feel examined, knowing how carefully I'm scrutinizing her bare backside. Down the fabric comes, slipping down over her cheeks and then down her legs, until I let them come to rest at mid-thigh.

And then I have her kneel down in the tub, and I watch as she does it, watch as she puts her head down and lifts her bottom up. I sit back down on the side of the tub, and Vaseline the nozzle and tell her that it has to go in her behind. I have her turn her head to watch as I Vaseline it. And then I reach out with one hand and spread her cheeks, making her wait for a minute like that before I put the tip of the nozzle against her rectum. I make her wait a bit longer , and then I begin to push the nozzle into her behind.

It goes in slowly, and I watch as it disappears between her spread cheeks, her behind slowly swallowing it. I watch her body to see how she's reacting to this slow penetration. Finally it's all in, I tell her that it's time. And I reach for the clamp on the hose.

✳ ✳ ✳

Apart from the bathtub the room is pretty usual, a toilet, a sink, a laundry basket in one corner. I walk to the sink and look at my reflection in the mirror; what I see is hardly shocking, hardly bestial. An ordinary enough man, an ordinary enough face, nothing out of the ordinary in the eyes.

I pull on the mirror to reveal the medicine cabinet behind it, and again there's nothing out of the ordinary there. The usual pills and potions, lotions and salves. What exactly am I looking for? I don't know.

There must be something, though. Some secret place. I'm not a policeman, but I take a cop's approach to her surroundings; there must be something that will reveal her to me, something covert that will open the door to her innermost thoughts. Evidence of her desires, insights into her innermost thoughts.

I close the medicine cabinet door and reach down and open the cabinet underneath the sink. A small plastic trashcan, empty. To its right, tile cleaner. Abrasive, sponges, all the usual cleaning supplies. I can see the rolls of toilet paper behind; nothing out of the ordinary, everything in its place. Which doesn't feel right to me somehow, so I take the trashcan out, and move the toilet paper. And behind it I see a plain box, pushed all the way to the back of the cabinet.

I pull it out and open it. Inside is an enema bag, a rectal plug, and a large jar of Vasline. I open the jar, and see that it's half empty, that there's a crater in the center where a nozzle has been dipped, many times.

I close the jar. Suddenly, I have a much better insight into her state of mind, and what she's been doing to prepare herself for my visit.

✳   ✳   ✳

It makes sense, of course, her preparation. In my fantasies I think about what she's feeling, what she thinks. "What will it feel like, the enema?" she must wonder, and I know she'll realize she doesn't have to wait for me to find out. And so I imagine her working up her courage to go to a drugstore and buy one, a combination bag, hot water bottle/douche/bag enema. How long does she fret about it, how long does it take her to work up the nerve? Lying in bed at night touching herself as she thinks about it, wonders what it will feel like, night after night climaxing to those fantasies, until she finally can't take it anymore.

On the day she goes to the drugstore, what does she feel, how does she dress? Does she masturbate before she goes, does she masturbate after? In the store she has that feeling in the pit of her stomach as she walks down the aisles to where the bags are kept, a place she knows well from previous trips. Does she blush when other customers walk by? Does she imagine them scrutinizing her, seeing into her soul, seeing her desires, seeing her guilt at what it is she knows she wants, knows she needs? Does she blush as she imagines them seeing her at home, kneeling in the tub, rear up with the nozzle in it?

She goes to the shelf where she knows she'll find it, scoops it quickly into her cart and then conceals it with other purchases. At the register she hangs back, trying to pick the least threatening cashier. A woman, she thinks, will be less intimidating than a man, but when it's her turn with the clerk — an indifferent teenager, gum chewing, unaware of her surroundings — she still feels as if the spotlight is on her. She feels the eyes of the older man behind her scrutinizing her purchases: soap, aspirins, other odds and ends; and then the combination bag.

There's no price on it, and the barcode isn't recognized by her register. "Price check, register 13," the girl calls into the microphone, and she stands there, mortified, until a manager comes to question the girl, to inspect the suspect merchandise. He holds it up to examine it, and now the whole line sees what it is. Oddly (but then this is my fantasy so nothing is odd; that's the ground rule of erotic fiction, anything that you want to be true, miraculously, is), no one seems to notice the hot water bottle use of the apparatus; she knows everyone sees the word "douche," though, and somehow "enema" glows in hot pink letters in their eyes.

After what seems like forever she finally escapes from the drugstore, her purchase in her bag. She will go elsewhere for the Vaseline; the rectal plug arrived in the mail that morning.

And when she's finally back in her house, she goes to her bedroom, and takes out the apparatus. Her hands shake a little as she sits and looks at it, but she is very excited, acutely aware of her backside on the cold rim of the large bathtub. She thinks about what's been arranged, thinks about me, although she doesn't really know me except by reputation. But in most ways that lack of knowledge is even more exciting. She wants it all to be unexpected. When will it happen? She doesn't know. What I will do she knows only in the most threadbare way; in fact there is no guarantee I will even keep her in her house for it, although, if I stay in character I will, because the Bandit himself never took a girl away from her apartment for the procedure he performed.

It's my fantasy, but I've known enough women to know that, in reality, she has been thinking about me, wondering what I'm like. Not just the physical details of what I look like, but how I act. How I sound when I talk: is my voice slow and comforting, harsh when she fails to obey? She must wonder what I sound like and what I'm going to say.

"Please take your pants down now," is that what it will be when it's time? Or something else, more intimate, "I'm going to take your pants down." Or, harsh: "Take your pants down; it's time." There are so many permutations, each a window into a different soul, and she knows me only from my writing and from the reassurances of her friend.

And now that I've seen the contents of the box under the sink, I know she's connected the two, the physical acts with the wonder of what I'm like and what I will do. I know that because of the plug; it's something the Bandit never did, but that we've agreed might happen. Bottom sex. Sodomy. A buggering. Or, in the crudest but most powerful way it can be described, "ass fucking."

I wonder which of the phrases she uses as she masturbates at night, as she finds her hands slipping between her legs in the early morning before work. I have my own fantasies on the matter; I think the one I like the best is that she thinks about my giving her "a good hard ass fucking, hard and deep."

But that's only my fantasy. I wonder which is hers.

❋   ❋   ❋

I realize that time has passed, and that I've seen all of the interior of her house I need to see, so I close the box containing the bag enema and the plug and put it back in its hiding place at the back of the sink. I put back the contents of the cabinet and close the doors. And I walk out of her room and back downstairs to the kitchen to get the big canvas bag that I've brought in with me but left there for safekeeping.

I look inside to see if I have everything I need, and I wonder for a moment if the Bandit did this too, and if so, when? Was it before he left his house, or apartment or wherever he stayed when he was committing his crimes? Was it in his car, after he'd picked the targets, made the decision and was about to act on it? Or did he wait, as I have, until he was inside?

I can't help but think about him and what he did, and it's both a disturbing and exciting thought. I don't condone it, but it excites me even so. As I walk from her kitchen upstairs to her bedroom, I know full well that I could never be here if it weren't prearranged, that I couldn't even enjoy the thought of it if it weren't agreed upon. But since it is, I've given my imagination free rein and I wonder often what he did, and how he did it.

I wonder what it would be like to give enemas to five girls in one evening; and then I try to think about how many people I've dealt with in one night, under *any* circumstances. Certainly more than one. More than two? Yes of course, but I have to think a while to recall the exact number, and when it comes to me I smile at the recollection it brings with it. Not of a cramped closet and unsuspecting prey; no, previous circumstances have been both more comfortable and less edgy. Pleasant circumstances, pleasant in their own way. A way very different from what's happening tonight.

Which is edgy, I won't deny it. Edgy for her, edgy for me, even with all my previous experiences. She's been preparing herself, and so have I, thinking and rethinking every enema I've given, reading the reports of the Bandit's activities and trying to combine the two, to put myself into his shoes, to the extent that I want to anyway. It's an odd kind of method acting, but not exactly an extrapolation. I've been allowing myself to slip into that role, the man who gave five coeds enemas on one night, allowing myself to feel the emotions I imagine he must have felt.

And what would those emotions have been? The first thing I imagine him feeling is sexual arousal. I always feel that, even when the enema is being given for disciplinary reasons alone. It turns me on to do it, after all, and the excitement starts when I see a woman walking down the street — any woman — and imagine her bare bottom with the hose in it and my hand on the clamp. Part of it is just that physical thing, the plain physical pleasure that comes from seeing a woman's bare backside, from feeling my hand on her warm supple skin and feeling it moving beneath my hand as I pull her cheeks apart and see between them. The physical feeling I get as I place the tip of the nozzle against her tight little opening and push it in.

But that's only the beginning. I think another big part of it is guessing what she's feeling, what she's thinking, how she's responding to everything I do. I'm pretty perceptive anyway, and if you've done it as many times as I have you see common responses you can use as milestones to your progress. But even without the squirming and the pleas, even without the body language that tells me what she's feeling, I know the sensations she's experiencing. The feeling of the nozzle, intrusive. And the enema, filling her. Her bowels expanding as the solution flows in.

I imagine that the Bandit's excitement must have started when he knew he was going to give one. That's what I feel, even if I don't have anyone in particular in mind yet. I know that it's *time*, and that once I've made the decision I'll find someone soon enough. I feel it from the top of my head to the tips of my toes. I've felt that way for years, about enemas, about spankings, and all the people I've talked to experience the same reaction. "I'm going to give you a spanking," I say, and the culprit reacts, the excitement spreads throughout the body, no matter how close or how far the spanking is from happening.

And then after I've absorbed that initial excitement, my next thought is who it's going to be, the recipient. Suddenly the behind of the woman at the next table takes on new significance, suddenly the skirt-covered backside of the girl leaning over at the counter captivates me in a way it didn't before. Suddenly a new erotic potential exists that wasn't there moments earlier, and I can follow that potential for hours, drifting along on it, fixating on this rump or that one, with no special need to single out any one at this point.

Now of course, unlike the Bandit, what I do is consensual, so after I know I'm going to give one, I have to find someone who will agree to what's going to happen. I can't just pick someone the way the Bandit did — I wouldn't want to — instead, I have to let her agree to being picked.

And how do I get someone to agree to taking an enema, erotic, disciplinary, whatever it is? I have to convince her, of course. I have to work at it, embark on a journey through her mind, leading her from refusal to downright capitulation, since I won't use force to bring her to that point. For me, nothing so crude — nothing so unexciting — as brute force. I use subtler tools. My aim is nothing less than her collusion in her submission. If I wanted someone on her knees, I'd guide her there on a path she follows of her *own* accord; she'll kneel because *she* wants her to, not because I forced her. And my pleasure comes in knowing that what I've offered up is so inviting that she'll follow of her own accord. And what could be more exciting than that?

And that makes me think about the box under the sink and what's in it. I realize that I have this woman captivated, and that turns me on. I've never met her, and yet I know all she thinks about is me. I know she thinks about me during the day. I know she masturbates when she gets home, and I'm pretty sure I can guess how she does it, too. I'm sure she's used that enema bag before, and after she's taken the solution she's pushed the plug into her ass thinking about me fucking her there. That's something she's thought about a lot, I'm sure of it; and after all, I've thought about it a lot too.

I'm sure she thinks about meeting me, and she thinks about that meeting as she wanders through every room of her house. Thinking about being spanked, thinking about being given an enema. If she were reading this now, she'd have the overwhelming desire to do everything I describe. To practice doing it. Not because I'm using force to get her to capitulate; no, her submission comes out of her own desires, and my only talent is to feed those desires. So there's no ego on my part in knowing she thinks about me. It doesn't make me feel bloated with pride or self-importance. Mostly it just turns me on to be able to bring someone so much pleasure without even having met in the flesh.

Why did she buy that enema bag and the rectal plug? To get ready for what I've made her want, to get ready for *me*, and I take pride in knowing that I've played so much of a role in it all. Every night she lies in bed and masturbates thinking about what's coming. Sometimes she takes an enema, sometimes she uses just the plug. On her knees, head down and bottom up, reaching back and pulling her cheeks apart, imagining it's me doing it. Imagining her cheeks are sore, and that she sees me Vaselining my cock as she spreads herself open for me. Sometimes she takes an enema and thinks about me doing it, punishing her with one, giving her one just because it pleases me. Giving her one because, after all, I'm playing the role of the Enema Bandit.

And that statement brings me out of my reverie there in the kitchen, and I look up at the clock and realize that it's time to get moving upstairs. So I hoist the bag onto my shoulder, go up the staircase and back to her bedroom, shutting the door to leave the house looking completely undisturbed.

I open the door to her closet, walk inside and close it behind me. I settle myself down in a back corner, moving clothes and boxes so that I won't be visible if she opens the door. I'm relatively comfortable here, and if I lean forward I can see out into her room through the open crack I've left. It reminds me so much of the vantagepoint I've written about in my stories; this time, it's real. Well, nothing to do now but wait.

I look at my watch. I have just enough time to collect myself before she gets home.

At any moment I expect to hear her car pulling into the driveway.

❋ ❋ ❋

As I wait I think about my fantasies leading up to this night, fantasies where I am the Bandit, perhaps even more so than the original Bandit might have allowed. I'm the Bandit, a Bandit of my own choosing, with a particular set of desires and plans that are different from those of the genuine article. So I spend a lot of my time thinking about things the Bandit never did, never saw.

As I sit in the quiet darkness of the closet I think about watching as she undresses and gets into bed. And about what she's going to do. Even before I found the box underneath the sink I thought about that, and the box only makes the fantasy stronger. So in my imagination I watch from the closet as she undresses and gets into bed. The lights are low and I can barely see her, but I hear her shifting as the minutes tick by. I listen, waiting for her breathing to settle as she slips off into sleep, but it doesn't happen. Something is keeping her awake as she lies there, something is keeping her from slumber.

I imagine seeing the light come on, watching her get out of bed, heading towards her bathroom. A late-night emptying of the bladder, I think, and indeed I hear the telltale sounds, and then the toilet flush and the sudden rush of water into the sink as she washes her hands. A long pause, and then I hear a cabinet opening. And finally she comes back out of the bathroom and back to her bed, carrying something in her hands. Now that I've been in her house, I know what it is that I only fantasized about before; it's the box with the plug and bag enema, of course, and she's looking at it as she sits down at the side of her bed, the beside lamp illuminating her face, the excitement I can read in her expression quite apparent.

And I watch from the closet as she opens the box, and takes out the enema bag and the jar of Vaseline. She does it in slow motion, as if she's rehearsing her actions. Or is it that she's imagining me doing it, with her watching from her tummy on the bed while I prepare it?

She takes out the bag, and holds it, turns it over and over in her hands, scrutinizes it, and then turns her attention to the long rubber hose and the nozzle on the end. She holds the nozzle in her hands, running her small fingers up and down the thick nozzle of ridged plastic, feeling the ridges, thinking about how it feels when it slides into her behind as she kneels on her bed with her head down. For a long time she holds the nozzle, as if she's watching me holding it, as if she's hearing me scolding her, chiding her, telling her what's about to come. As if she's working up her resolve. And then she suddenly stands up, and faces the bed. Puts her hands in the waistband of her pajamas and slowly — agonizingly slowly — pulls them down to her knees.

I watch as the pajamas descend, revealing the two rounded moons of her behind and the darkly shaded crack that separates them. Down her pajamas come, down the fabric goes, slowly revealing her rump, a curtain falling, a slow striptease just for me. I imagine the vulnerability she'll feel when she does it in front of me, knowing what's coming next. Seeing the thick nozzle stiff in my hands, knowing something thicker and stiffer still lies in wait in my pants.

And then, when her pajamas are at her knees, I watch her climb up onto her bed, her cheeks parting as she puts one knee on the bed and pushes herself up. Soon she is kneeling there, her head down, her bottom high. The pajama bottoms at mid-thigh and the top coming down to just below her waist, a frame for the "target." She reaches for the Vaseline and begins to lubricate the nozzle as I watch. And then she shuffles her knees as far apart as the pajama bottoms will allow and puts the head of the nozzle against her rectum. For some reason she's turned her head to the side that faces me as she holds the nozzle there, and I can see her face tensing as she works up her courage. I watch her teasing her anus with the tip of the nozzle, tickling herself with it as she presses it in, pausing a moment before allowing it to fully penetrate her.

As I watch this scene in my mind I imagine sensing a smell, a warm musty smell of arousal, and I know that, although the room is too dark for me to see it, there's a wet patch growing between her legs as she caresses her rectum with the nozzle. I wonder if she's ever been penetrated there before by anything other than the nozzle and the rectal plug she keeps in the box. Will my latex-clad cock be the first to plumb that dark, tight, forbidden passageway to pleasure? Will I be the first to spread her cheeks and thrust myself into that warm Vaselined passage? Will I be the first to look down and see her upthrust ass, her red cheeks spread around my cock as I fuck her there? Will I be the first to fuck her backside, the first to fuck her ass? I hope I will be.

And as I think about that I imagine watching her slowly pushing the nozzle in, watching the thick white tube disappear up her behind. I hear her moaning now, a soft low moan that gets louder and more plaintive as the tube goes in. Louder and louder it gets, the sound growing, swelling as she masturbates in front of me, head down on her bed, her bottom up high with the nozzle in her rear.

Louder and louder, and then — suddenly — I realize that it's not my fantasy, that noise. It's the sound of a car pulling into her driveway.

She's coming home. In a few minutes she'll be inside the house.

❄ ❄ ❄

I hide in her closet upstairs in her room as I listen to her come into her house. I hear her walking into the kitchen, the rustle of packages, the thump of the refrigerator door. Soon I hear her coming out into her living room, and the TV goes on. I hear the downstairs toilet flush, and I know she's on the couch watching TV.

What is she thinking? She knows I could be upstairs, is that why she hasn't come up yet to change out of her work clothes? Is her mind on the evening news, the parade of nightly gore? Or is it on her room, on her closet perhaps, and who might be hiding there, waiting for her? Is she downstairs because she has no reason to come up yet — or is it because she's afraid to, because she has to work up her courage to what she knows might be up here? Me. That's what might be up here, me, hiding in her closet waiting for her.

For a long time I listen to her downstairs, first watching TV and then, from the noises I hear in the kitchen, cooking a quick frozen dinner. She's downstairs, and I'm upstairs, and the physical gap that bridges us is small, but the emotional one she must be feeling is vast. She's coming to terms with it, I think, putting herself in the right frame of mind. Perhaps imagining she's one of those coeds on that fateful night, the night the Bandit struck. Whatever it is, I'm waiting for her to finish, to come upstairs to where I'm waiting.

And eventually she does. I hear the TV go silent, I hear her footsteps into the kitchen, the sound of washing dishes. I hear her back out in the living room now, straightening, and then I hear her footsteps moving across the room to the stairwell.

I hear each step on each tread, or at least I think I do. Left foot. Right foot. Left foot, right foot, and I hear her pause on the landing, and I know it's not a shortage of breath that's making her wait there but the fear in her guts. The butterflies in her tummy at what might be upstairs in the dark. I hear her pause. And then I hear her footsteps again, coming down the hallway to her bedroom door.

The sound of the lock turning, and I hear that low whisper as the bottom of the door glides across the thick carpeting of her room. I can almost feel the slight change in air pressure as she walks inside, and I am holding my breath now as I hear her feet walk towards me, towards the closet. I hold my breath, waiting for the door to open… and then I exhale silently when I hear a thump outside the door and realize it's a pile of clothes that she's dropped there. I hear her go to her dresser, hear the drawers opening, and I know it's clothes she's dropped outside the closet, and that she's changing now into something more comfortable.

The water runs in her bathroom as she brushes her teeth, and then I hear the door shut with a bang. Who closes the bathroom door when they're alone in their own house? Force of habit? Or does she think I might be there, is she seeking privacy from the possibility of my gaze? I hear the bathroom door close and, eventually, I hear the sound of the toilet flushing, the sound of water in the sink as she washes her hands.

I hear the sound of a cabinet being opened — the one over the sink or the one under it? — and a long silence. Faint rustling noises, and now the cabinet door closing again. I hold my breath, this time in anticipation, and as I keep myself from breathing I inch forward until my eye is at the crack in the closet door.

I can see the room, the lamp on by the bed, the low illumination throwing fearsome shadows into the corners. I see the outline of the bathroom door, and I wonder what she's doing inside. The outline goes dark, and I see the door opening.

She's coming out now, wearing white pajamas, matching top and bottom, white socks on her feet. It's too dark to see her at first, but as she comes closer to her bed, I see she's holding something in her hands.

It's the box from underneath her sink. It's open.

And as she tips it forward under the light from her bedside lamp I see she has the jar of Vaseline uncovered. And her hand is on the thick plastic enema nozzle.

She gets into bed. I lean forward and press my eye tighter to the crack in the closet door to see what she'll do next.

❄ ❄ ❄

And, for all my experience, what she does now surprises me. No, floors me actually — I, who have seen it all, done it all, I thought I know what she would do.

But I realize I'm wrong; and the enormity of my mistake jumps out at me as she reaches over and picks up the phone by her bed, punches in a number and lies back against the pillows. She waits — we wait — for it to ring, and apparently it does for she begins speaking into it, the soft sultry tone of her voice immediately confirming my suspicions.

"I'm in my bedroom," she says, "and I've got my box in my hands. He might be coming tonight; he might be here now… what do you want me to do…?" As she speaks she settles back further into her pillows, and I watch her looking at the nozzle she holds in her hand, watch her cradle the phone against her shoulder, watch her slip her free hand down to the front of her pajamas, and then down inside them. I see her hand moving underneath the soft white fabric as she talks…

I don't know who it is she's talking to. Her boyfriend? A disciplinarian? I'm sure it's a man, but who it is eludes me, and I feel a momentary sense of frustration replaced instantly by anger. Anger that she should dilute her excitement with thoughts of someone else;

that she should ruin *our* moment with the participation of a third party. I feel that she's cheating on me somehow, I feel as if I'm just a pawn in a game she's playing, and I think I should just stay there until she's asleep and then leave. Leave, without letting her know I've been there at all. Or, better yet, leave her a note telling her that I know what she's been doing, and I want no part of it. None at all.

But then I find myself beginning to be excited by what I'm witnessing. He's not there, after all; and it's really only acting to build her anticipation about me, increasing my power, something I can't possibly find abhorrent. I'll just let her talk a while longer, I think, and then make the final decision about how I feel. So I let myself cool down somewhat, and keep my eye on her as I listen to what she's saying on the phone.

And she begins to talk to the man on the other end of the line, describing where she is and what she's wearing. She moves her hand in front as she talks, and I'm almost embarrassed at the intimacy of the moment I'm witnessing. A voyeur in her closet, watching her masturbate herself in front of me, without knowing I'm there. I've had plenty of culprits rub themselves before correction; and I've rubbed plenty more. This is different, somehow, with me in this position of concealment, watching her rub. Throughout the evening I've found myself in odd moral quandaries: how thorough an exploration of her house to make; how many of the letters in her box in her study should I read; should I really be there listening to her conversation now? Quandaries, but the thing is I'm hard now, very hard, and whatever residual morality I have at the moment is thoroughly overruled by that priapic principle. Tumescence trumps timidity. Each and every time.

I listen to her talking to him, and I watch as she puts the phone down so she can get both hands on her pajama bottoms. She rolls over onto her stomach first, puts both hands on the waistband and pulls them down, slowly. By random chance she's pointing her backside almost directly at me as she does so, and I watch her baring her behind, slowly. Recalling all the fantasies I've had about this moment. She pulls her pajama bottoms down, stopping when they're at her knees.

Her bottom is completely bared, and my eyes are fixated on it. I'm carrying the memory of the moment when she had to lift herself up on her knees slightly to get the pajamas down, and how her cheeks spread apart when she did so. A moment, a moment only, but I caught enough of a glimpse between her legs to know she's shaved down there; to see the glistening smoothness of her inner thighs and the bare folded fig that lies at the base.

The pajamas are down and she's picked up the phone again, and as she's talking she's holding the Vaselined nozzle in one hand, bringing it back towards her behind as she talks. I wonder if she's directing him, or if she's simply telling him what she thinks I'll be doing later; that night, or whatever night she thinks I might be there waiting for her. I can't figure it out but I don't suppose it matters much; what's she's doing is much more engrossing than who's running the show, and I watch quietly, intently, as she slips the nozzle into her behind, pushing back with her bottom to slowly take it up her ass.

She begins to move the nozzle in and out, and I hear her telling the guy on the other end of the phone what she's doing, I hear her say "I'm getting my ass fucked," over and over, and I can tell from how slowly she's moving the nozzle that she's enjoying the sensation terribly, that she's tightening her ass on the nozzle to get the maximum effect from the penetration.

She pushes the nozzle in and out of her ass, and I watch her, imagining it's my cock back there; and then she stops suddenly, and there's a long pause as she listens to what the man on the other end of the line is saying. I watch as she gets up off her bed, the nozzle still rudely protruding from her bare posterior. She waddles off towards the bathroom, her pajama bottoms at her knees, holding the empty enema bag high, the hose dangling down from the bottom of the bag, down to lowest point and then rising again, rising up to the thick white nozzle penetrating her ass.

She disappears into the bathroom, and closes the door, leaving me there in the closet hard — oh so very hard — staring at the phone on her bed wondering if the man on the other end is as hard as I am. For a long time she's in the bathroom, and I hear the water running in the sink, and I know what she's doing, I know it perfectly well even before she comes back out, pajamas still down, bag still high — this time, completely filled. Back to the bed she goes, where she picks up the phone again and then shuffles off to the corner, where I notice there's a stool.

I wonder how many nights she's been doing this. I wonder at that as I see her hanging the bag from a hook in the wall I hadn't noticed before, see her bending over the stool, watch her cheeks flexing apart as she bends. Watch her pajama bottoms slipping down her legs, see her two white bare cheeks with the nozzle spearing between them. She holds the phone in her left hand; with her right she reaches back and begins to fuck her ass with the nozzle, this time pulling it completely out and pausing a moment before she pushes it back in. She's pushing her weight down onto the stool as she does this, and I realize there's a reason for that: she's rubbing herself against the stool, bringing herself off as she gets her ass fucked and talks to her friend on the phone.

Over and over I watch the nozzle going in and out, and I listen to what she's saying. She's talking about the Bandit, and the five coeds, and how she's going to be the sixth; only *her* bandit is going to fuck her ass after he's washed it out. He's going to clean her ass and then put her over the stool for a bottoms-up-cheeks-apart, and he's going to take his belt off and give her the strap if she doesn't behave herself while she's getting it.

Over and over I watch the nozzle going in and out, and I'm throbbing in synchrony with the motions of the nozzle; as it pushes in I can actually feel the tightness of her rectum sliding over the head of my cock. I watch, I hear her moan, and I see her hand moving now, up from the nozzle to grasp the clamp on the hose. And I hear her telling the guy on the phone that she feels it getting bigger in her ass and that she's about to get a sperm enema, and I watch her hand inching up to the clamp as she says that and I can tell she's getting near to orgasm. Totally lost in her own little world, thinking only of what she feels, lost except for the sensations she feels and the sensation she's about to feel, that soapy water shooting up her behind as she masturbates over the stool with her friend on the other end of the line listening.

Suddenly, I realize it's time. And I slide the closet door open, so quietly I know she doesn't hear, and I walk out of the closet towards her, and she's too lost in her own passion to notice.

And I come up behind her, look down at her bare bottom with the nozzle in it and her hand inching up to the clamp.

And I reach out and put *my* hand on the clamp, and just as her hand slides up to reach mine and the sudden realization of my being there hits her, I open it with a loud *click*.

As the water hits her bowels, as the soapy enema shoots deep into her suddenly resistant backside, she has an orgasm.

The first of several she'll have that evening.

Oh, and by the way, there never was anyone on the other end of the line. She did all that for me, on the assumption that I might be there, watching.

A very sexy lady indeed.

A PHILLIPIC ON MORALITY

Yes, there is such a thing as morality. And yes, it applies to everything I've described in this book (I certainly hope that the reader is clear by now that some of the stories contained herein are fantasies, and intended to be read as such). I want to make these two points clear because non-judgmentalism and the deconstruction of ideas and cultural imperalism notwithstanding, underneath it all there are still things that are *right*, and things that are *wrong*. And I'm going to address them, here and now.

---

1.   *Children and Young Adults (Teens)*

A child is the most wonderful thing in the world, and the slightest unhappiness on an adult's part with a child's behavior is something so fundamentally distressing to a child that any other measures, especially physical ones, are not just brutal: they're *wrong*. So let me make it clear: *nothing* in this book, and I do mean *nothing*, should *ever* be applied to children. Unless it's the idea that everyone deserves respect and fair treatment, children included. And just to make it completely clear, when you read the appellation "Daddy" in the text, that should never be taken to be a statement of biological relatedness; it isn't. It's a term of respect and endearment. A statement that one person looks up to the other as a father, and that the other wishes to show all the tenderness and care that a good father shows his offspring.

Now let's talk about young adults, i.e. teenagers, below the age of consent. It would be a canard to say or even to think that teens are not sexually active or present on the Internet, whether pretending to be older or, more than likely, giving their real ages to adults who find that youth even more enthralling. And I have two words for adults who wish to pursue relationships with such teens: *illegal* and *immoral*.

Let's talk about *illegal* first; it's so much easier to grasp abstract philosophical concepts that, in Lewis Carroll's pungent words, have "the jaws that bite, the teeth that catch." So in case you didn't know — if for example you were Rip van Winkle — having sex with someone under the age of 18 (or the age of consent in your state — if you're not sure, check *www.ageofconsent.com*) is illegal, as is meeting them for that purpose, even in the absence of the act itself. The consequence is criminal prosecution. *Criminal prosecution.* Time in jail. Certainly your face and name on the front page of your local newspaper, the destruction of your family, etc. Do I have to make it clearer than that?

Moreover, it's *immoral*. I'm not a fan of Dr. Laura; in fact I detest the kind of pat "morality" she appears to espouse. But there's a reason why people below the age of consent are protected by these kinds of laws, and it has to do with the ability to consent. Now I won't claim that the day he or she turns adult Dick or Jane suddenly becomes immune from the suggestibility that characterizes youths. Hardly; there are people in their 70s who are suggestible, and 10-year-olds who are the most hardened skeptics I've ever encountered. But the basic idea — the basic moral principle — is that there be consent to the acts I've described, and someone under the age of consent is far too susceptible to undue influence to be counted on to give consent.

In case that wasn't clear the first time around, let me reword it; everything I've described is consensual, and someone under the age of consent certainly can't give consent the way someone older can. You can badger someone into saying yes, you can convince them it's what they want, and maybe it is in whatever abstract epistemological way that such questions can be answered. But the lesson I'm preaching is that "yes" can't be taken to mean "yes" when the person saying it is under the age of consent.

So do yourself and that person a favor: stay away from people under the age of consent. And if you're under the age of consent, wait. As I said I'm not sure that any magic happens on that special birthday, but at least it's something. At least there's some hope of consensuality with someone of age.

2.   *Consensuality; or "If you were really submissive ..."*

Enlarging on the previous discussion of the consensual nature of all of this, let's consider the paradigm example of the mental bludgeoning that occurs every day in hundreds if not thousands of conversations about dominance and submission: "If you were *really* submissive you would have done what I asked you to do ..."

That statement is probably the single *most* immoral statement that can ever be delivered in a dominant/submissive relationship; immoral because it totally annihilates consent. Consider what it means, really, what it says in translation. Do you know what that is? It's this: "I wanted you to do something, and you didn't do it. So I'm going to fuck with your head and make you feel that there's something wrong with *you* for not doing what I want, rather than allowing us to talk about it as two sympathetic human beings to find out if there was something wrong with *me* for having demanded you do something that you weren't ready to do. Or quite possibly will never be able to do at all."

It obviates consent because it makes someone feel guilty for not instantly capitulating. Not even guilty, because that's far too mild an encapsulation: guilty, inadequate, a failure, disobedient, a smorgasbord of shortcomings. And it's immoral because consensuality is such a tenuous concept under any circumstance.

Here's the bottom line. If you are the dominant, it is your *responsibility* not to use statements like this; it is your *responsibility* to seek to understand whether what you want is reasonable, and whether the person you are dominating is not giving you what you want because it's wrong of you to want it in the first place. In case it had never occurred to you, you see, it's not okay for you to have everything you want.

And if you are the submissive, it's *your* responsibility to understand that a statement like "If you were *really* submissive ..." should register in your mind the way the matador's red cape does in the mind of the bull; it should enrage you, make you angry, make you want to charge. Because it's almost always a shitty thing to say; it's an accusation that there's something wrong with you for not giving the other person anything he or she wants. And the truth is that, maybe you are in the wrong, but equally there's no reason to think that the relationship consists simply of you giving the other person everything.

---

3.   *Consensuality: it's okay to say "NO!" to some things*

To continue the previous discussion, it's perfectly okay to say *no!* to doing some things, and that means both from the dominant's and the submissive's point of view. If you go to a bar and find yourself talking to someone who is perfect in every way except that he/she loves country music, or Republicans, or Democrats, or mud-wrestling, or Emeril Lagasse, then you both have to accept that perhaps you have no business being together or, if you do try to make a go of it, that some things can't safely be done.

Consensual relationships are based on the same under-standing: that some things have to be off-limits because they don't work for one of the parties. And quite honestly, if there are enough things off-limits perhaps you are both better off finding other people to explore your feelings with. For example, although I like to introduce people initially resistant to enemas and other anal activities to the realm of my experiences, I am very up-front about the fact that what I do isn't for everyone, nor should it be. I will encourage, but I will not demand; I make it a simple fact that, in a relationship with me, enemas and other anal activities will occur, and I encourage the person I'm talking to to consider whether or not that's what they want. If it isn't, that's fine. It means they need to find someone other than me. The more you find yourself selling your own charms to an uncertain audience — or the more you find yourself listening to someone offering a hard pitch — the more you should realize that what's going on has more to do with desire than with respect. And respect is what it's all about.

4. *Team Sports; or, the natural order of things.*

A further extension of consensuality is what happens as a relationship evolves. One aspect is what I will call "team sports," meaning the involvement of other people in what had previously been a one-on-one interaction.

My feeling is that there is nothing wrong with the introduction of new people into a relationship, as long as both parties are comfortable with what those people will see and how they will fit in. That is, as long as both parties have communicated what they want and seen their wishes heard and respected.

Which is the primary point of this section: communication and respect. All relationships evolve, and things that at one point would have been inconceivable often become irresistible with time. But there's a natural progression to be observed, a gradual one, with respect and trust preserved — magnified — at each step. So keep in mind that the natural order of things is that small steps lead to big steps. Cast in the "If you were really submissive you would have done what I asked you to do ..." argument, one correct response to this sort of statement is to say, "I may be able to do what you want. I'd like to... but things have to move more slowly." Remember, it's okay to ask for that, that things go slowly. And, for the dominant, it's okay to make them go slowly even when the submissive wants them to go fast.

5. *Crying*

For many people, crying seems to be the sought-after endpoint of a discipline session; "will I cry?" is a question that I'm almost always asked when I describe how I discipline.

So let's talk about crying, what it means to cry and how crying can be appropriately achieved. First of all, what does it mean to cry?

Under the right circumstances, crying represents catharsis, emotional release expressed in physical form. Crying of this sort is profound; a gift, one that should be honored, one that should be treasured. The person crying should be held, comforted, help to recover his or her equilibrium after being taken to that place of release by the disciplinarian. That's not optional behavior for the disciplinarian: the disciplinarian *must* care for the culprit after this sort of release. Failure to do so is immoral, plain and simple.

The problem with crying is that it can be made to occur for the wrong reasons. Basically emotional abuse can get someone to cry — but that's not a release, it's a breaking down of someone, which I don't see as a positive thing at all. As an example, consider yelling at someone, calling him or her dirt and making biting accusations all of which are true enough to hurt, hard enough to bite, and to continue doing that until the person weeps. Is that crying? Yes. Is there anything positive about it? No. Because where's the catharsis? Where's the building up that follows the tearing down?

I'm sure that some readers will disagree; I know that in some schools of BDSM tearing down is seen as a prerequisite to rebuilding in the mold the creator sets. I'm sorry, but I have trouble believing this, probably because I think that only God has the right to make man or woman in his image — and most of the men and women I've seen in the scene are on a distinctly earthy and not ethereal plane (myself included).

So my take on it is that the goal should never be getting someone to cry, because with that as the endpoint it's far to easy to use the wrong set of emotional tools (abusive ones), and then, having achieved the crying, walk away thinking either that you've done a great job ("I'm a wonderful dom because, as I said, when we meet, you *will* cry") or, having cried, walk away thinking that crying you just did must have been a great experience even though you feel like shit.

Crying doesn't happen in every meeting; and someone who says that it does is, more than likely, using a set of tools that cause distress, not release. I'm sure that some readers disagree. But I have yet to be convinced that the statements I'm making are anything but true.

6.   *Sex and Discipline*

Finally, discipline and sex. Discipline and sex are closely allied; scene and sex are closely allied; but what I've described in this book is not just about sex. To many dominants, what they do boils down to getting sex, and the kind that they like. My advice to submissives is, if you find yourself in a relationship where you have sex but don't have your emotional needs addressed, the person you are dealing with is practicing sex, not dominance. If that works for you, fine, but don't confuse one with the other. As I hope I've made clear in what I've written, the experience is so much more than sexual; it includes arousal, but it reaches beyond to the emotions, to feelings. To all the things that make true sexuality — the combination of penetration, sensation, emotion, friendship, respect — such a heady thing.

THE REORIENTATION

At 4:30 am the phone begins ringing, loudly and insistently.

The young man in the bed stirs, reaching his arm out to find the receiver, groping for a minute on the nightstand. The arm moves to the left, then the right, knocking an opened book off the crowded wood surface and onto the cold hardwood floor, where it lands with a dull thud. Back to the right, and then across until his hand passes over the cool plastic of the phone. A pause, the hand descends, grips the phone and hoists it up from the receiver.

The muscular arm withdraws from the table, phone in hand, disappearing slowly under the thick pile of blankets, sleepily cradling it to his ear.

"Hello …" he says groggily, half-awake in the cold of early morning, hours away from the sun.

"Hank Jones?" The voice on the other end of the line is unfamiliar, but has the same hardness and efficiency as the other unknown and uninvited voices he's been subjected to over the last two weeks, the two weeks of misery and anticipation since the ticket. The voice snaps him awake, instantly. He blurts out a quick, husky, uncertain "Yes…?"

There's a pause, and the faint sound of papers being rustled, the sharp clicking of a computer keyboard. "Hank," the unfamiliar voice speaking too personally, too intimately, full of masked menace and condescension. "It seems there's been an unexpected… vacancy… in the reorientation program you were informed about in your sentencing letter…"

More clicking, and the sound of a supervisor being consulted *in sotto voce*. He is clutching the phone to his ear, sweating now, feeling his stomach in knots, hearing the occasional *whoosh* of a lone car passing on the cold dark deserted street below his apartment.

"We've reserved that spot for you, Hank. You've been scheduled for initial processing this morning. Seven a.m. – the car will be there by six. There will be a nurse to select the things you'll need for your stay. Review the instructions given in the letter if you have any questions..."

A long pause, and he slowly becomes aware of a muted *thud thud thud*, a sound that slowly resolves itself into his own heartbeat, the fist-sized ball of muscle dancing a heavy jig in his pounding chest. He continues to clutch the phone, stupidly, dazed. Only gradually realizing that the line has gone dead, that the unfamiliar but overly friendly voice on the other end has concluded its business and hung up. Gone on to its next victim perhaps, some other young man startled awake in the pre-dawn to have his sentence calmly and indifferently announced.

Under the covers now, deep in the cocooning warmth, he experiences a momentary mirage. Sees his foot lifting up off the pedal moments before he passes the spot where the police car lies in wait. Sees himself looking down at the speedometer, sees the needle dipping down, dropping down, descending down into the safe zone. Sees himself waving amiably at the cop suddenly revealed. He glides by the black-and-white in wait, continues on into the bright circle of his undisturbed life stretching out at the end of the tunnel of tarmac.

The clock ticks, the mirage fades into a windswept, waterless desert of despair. Under the blankets he is suffocating now, remembering how he swept through the turn, how the police car roared out after him, lights flashing, sirens blaring.

He remembers the look in the burly cop's eyes as he stood there writing the ticket, and how the blood rushed to Hank's face when he looked down at it, thrust into his unwilling hand by the unsmiling cop, waiting for his signature.

Hank held the pen for a long moment above the pale surface, wandering from the blank line where he would write his name to the lines above where his crime had been recorded. "Speed limit... 50." "Clocked speed... 75." 25 miles an hour difference, and he sat in the car with the number dancing in his head as his buttocks tightened in his well-worn denim jeans.

His throat tightened as he signed it, recalling Casey, his older friend. Casey, who had been pale and silent the day he finally was allowed back to work. Casey, that day and every day for the next week, standing, when others sat. Leaving for lunchtime appointments at the station house in the company of a warden, while his coworkers sat and watched, and ate in undisturbed bliss.

Casey, returning at the end of each lunch hour, walking slowly into the office, slowly back to his desk. Standing there erect, his eyes red-rimmed, red indentations still plainly apparent around his hairy wrists where the handcuffs had been.

Hank is breathing hard now thinking about it, breathing hard as he climbs slowly out of the warm blankets into the cold air of the apartment. Labored breath as he turns on the shower and steps under its drenching spray. He stands there, naked, the water pressure turned up as high as it will go, thinking the unwanted thought that has tormented him day after day for the last two weeks.

Standing there, the water striking his chest, running down in a warm stream over his cold flesh, caressing his balls, his shriveled cock. He turns, letting the water sleet down onto his buttocks, feeling the individual droplets pelt one cheek, and then the other.

Standing there in the shower he recalls Casey's sentencing sheet, which he saw as he walked by the older man's desk. For each mile over the limit, 10 strokes with a leather strap.

Casey had been going 35 in a 25-mile-an-hour zone, and had suffered for a week, standing for a week in wincing pain, enduring the whispered comments of his coworkers and his daily escort to the station for other unknown and unspeakable horrors.

For each mile over the limit, 10 strokes with a leather strap. Casey had suffered through a hundred strokes.

Casey had gotten 100 strokes. Hank would receive 250.

As he steps from the shower, and reaches for the towel in the half-light, his doorbell rings.

His heart drops into his stomach, and from there down through the floor beneath him to the ground below.

✳ ✳ ✳

An older man stands calmly outside the opened door in the hallway, stands looking at Hank for a long moment. From head to toe. Not just looking, not even sizing him up the way men will do with other men. *Examining* him, as if he had been put under a microscope. Taking in each detail as his eyes travel slowly down, scanning the body inadequately concealed by the small towel around the hips. Down, over the slender shoulders to the chest, surprisingly hairy, muscles firm but still soft somehow, youthful. Slim hips, long legs, feet turning chilly on the cold morning floor.

The man shakes his head from side to side. "Body hair — that won't do at reorientation," he remarks casually, reaching into the bag he carries across his chest as he speaks.

He produces a thick booklet which he hands to Hank. "Not much *is* allowed without judge's orders... boy." He pushes the "b" out of his mouth as if he's spitting, the sound of a faint accent from the old South an undercurrent to his speech. "This tells you most of what you need to know."

Hank stares at it, dumbly, then up at man in front of him, taking him in for the first time. Tall, middle-aged, expressionless face, with featureless khakis and shirt to match. Only the black boots stand out as distinctive; polished to perfection, they gleam in the faint light.

They stand there for a moment, an odd pair. Hank is suddenly aware of his nakedness, at the inadequacy of the towel. It barely covers his ass, descends only a inch or so below his cock. He is virtually nude in front of this stranger.

The man gestures him into his apartment, and Hank turns, reluctantly and walks in.

The man follows, and Hank waits to hear the sound of his door being closed. It does not come. What he does hear as he slowly drags himself past his kitchen is the unpleasant sound of a neighbor's door opening, softly and slowly, but not enough to mask the telltale creak of the eavesdropper's un-oiled hinge.

A little too loudly, the man behind Hank says, "Into your bedroom." Hank obeys.

The orders continue, the voice still too loud. "Remove the towel. Good boy. Place it in the hamper. No, pick it up and put it inside.

That's right, bend all the way over to get it." Hank is mortified, wants to put his hands back behind him, but recognizes the inadvisability of that action.

"Good. Now get your cute little backside over the end of your bed, both hands on the sheets. And I don't have to tell you to keep them there..." At this point, Hank feels despair. The despair of being revealed, of having the sentence he has managed to hide from his neighbors for the last few weeks exposed suddenly. As thoroughly as if the police had passed through with a bullhorn or a sound truck and made his crime... and upcoming punishment... common knowledge.

Hank, a private person who has never said more than a sentence or two to any of his neighbors, now stands in shame at the end of his bed, the man behind him as Hank resigns himself to the inevitable. Bends forward, slowly leans down, places both hands on the sheets, still perceptibly warm with the heat of his own body.

He looks at his hands before him, tries not to the think what the man behind him sees — what the "nurse" sees, he corrects himself. His bare ass, the cheeks spread by his position, his muscular legs rising to the firm buttocks, evidence of the hours he spends at the gym. Firm buttocks, and in this position everything between them visible, the tight hole between. And, beneath them, the balls, retracted in the cold air, the cock shriveled too, although out of fear.

Hank waits, bending, knowing the nurse sees everything he has to offer.

Not by choice. But by the power of the law.

Images of Casey fill Hank's mind again. The buttocks tighten.

For the first time, the nurse's expression changes. A slight smile twists the corners of the mouth up.

In position, Hank isn't able to see it. And, if he did, it's not likely that he would find it comforting.

❋   ❋   ❋

As Hank waits, the nurse opens his bag, slowly unzipping it, reaching inside to withdraw something. Hank hears the loud *snap* of a rubber glove in the early morning stillness, the sound of a jar being unscrewed, and of a package being opened carefully and set down on the table nearest the nurse.

"We'll start by inserting the electronic monitoring device. Once I activate it, it will emit a loud squeal if it falls out... or if you're foolish enough to try to remove it yourself. It's shaped to stay in, but I brought along a retention belt if you don't think you have enough muscle control to grip it... do you want to authorize my using it?"

Hank screws his eyes tight, and gives a forlorn nod. The nurse approaches, monitoring device in one hand, the open container of Vaseline in the other.

"We'll need to get started then," he says, "and you can sign the consent form later. Now brace yourself against the bed and push back... and hold yourself *still* for me. This only takes a minute... I've been told that it doesn't hurt a bit..."

Hank's anus goes desperately tight as he hears the nurse's last words, hears them at the same time that he feels the thickly greased finger against him there, pushing against his tight ring. A small groan escapes his lips as the nurse applies pressure and his asshole begins to yield.

The enforced penetration has begun.

❋   ❋   ❋

Seven am, and a second khaki-clad man stands outside the driver's seat of his institutional-green bus, nondescript and unremarkable in every way but two: in large white letters on its side are the block-stenciled words "Department of Corrections (DOC) – Men"; and, there are surprisingly thick steel bars on the windows. Like the nurse, the DOC bus driver's khakis are shapeless, the black boots gleam, and there is no expression on the face. Despite the early morning hour, large sunglasses hide his eyes.

From his vantage point at the side of the bus the driver scans the empty parking lot, his eyes roving past the occasional parked car, oil-stained patch of pavement and broken beer bottle, remnant of a weekend's boisterous activities. His eyes narrow at the sight of the broken glass, and he makes a mental note to recommend increased weekend patrols in the area, imagining the police delivering up the miscreants to him as he does so. The last two he has dealt with for littering and drunken disorderliness screamed and moaned their way through their tandem canings, disgracing themselves in several other humiliating ways in the process. A faint smile crosses the man's face as he recalls the basement records of their correction, the sight of the stripped asses, and the shriveled testicles and cocks beneath. The videotaped apologies that accompany them. A source of much motivation to fresh admittees forced to study them at the intake and processing center. And useful material for young staff members as well, at least for those seeking to improve their work skills as a way of rising through the ranks.

❋ ❋ ❋

A flicker of activity at one end of the lot catches the driver's attention and interrupts his reverie, and his head catches in mid-turn, swivels back and locks onto the spot, his eyes following his targets as they slowly pick their way past the cars and bottles to the waiting bus.

Three men slowly approaching the car. The older man – the nurse – in the standard khakis of a DOC employee, the two younger men in street clothes. The nurse leads, the young men trail after him. Although the distance is too great to see expressions clearly, the driver waiting at his bus knows the looks on those two faces well, having seen similar ones hundreds if not thousands of times before during his many years in service.

Downturned mouths, sad eyes, probably already crying. Both men follow the nurse in what staff members have come to call the "intake shuffle," a slow unsteady walk, feet abnormally far apart, body tensed and slightly bent, buttocks protruding slightly. A gait that has always been a habit for new admittees, churning stomachs, tensing bowels, shrunken cocks at the prospect of what's about to happen to them. But, since the advent of the electronic monitoring devices that the DOC now uses to prevent escapes, the explanation for the intake walk has become considerably simpler.

After all, the driver thinks as the three cross the last ten feet of discolored concrete to stand in front of him, how easy can it be to walk with a rubber-coated metal plug six inches long and almost two inches in diameter locked tightly and securely into such a tight little hole?

❋ ❋ ❋

The bus driver smiles again, this time a distinctly unpleasant smile for the benefit of the admittees, looks up at the four other men already inside the bus staring out through the bars, and then down again at the clipboard in his hands. Four names checked off, three still to go.

"Right," he says, not looking up, "Wheeler… and *Jones*…" His hand moves deftly, two names checked, now only one line unmarked. He clips the pen to the board, looks up at the two cowering young men.

"Welcome to the DOC, boys. A most exclusive country club, and I'm *sure* you'll both be enjoying your stays."

He looks at the nurse, who nods his head. "They've both been activated?" he asks, and once again the nurse nods his ascent.

"Good," he says, pulling what looks to be a largish pager from his belt, lifting its plastic cover and scrutinizing the blinking lights inside. A bank of ten little bulbs, six flashing green, the remaining four unlit. He looks back up. "Well, boys, you're all on my monitor, and my chariot awaits, if you'd be so kind as to climb aboard. We only have one more stop to make."

He reaches up into the cab of the bus, pushes a button. The door to the rear section swings open, the faint hiss of air escaping the pneumatics audible through the still-quiet morning air. The two men climb up the stairs, slowly, in clear discomfort, and the door swings shut behind them.

The driver climbs in, the nurse walks around to the passenger's seat and sits down, looking back to make sure that the new wards of the state are all present and accounted for.

The driver starts the ignition, puts the bus into gear and slowly rolls it out of the parking lot, passing Hank's neighbors standing outside their cars, about to leave to start their normal workdays.

The faces of his neighbors are shocked and unsmiling as they recognize Hank sitting white-faced in the window, his forehead resting against the cold bars.

The bus pulls out of the lot and onto the street, turns south, towards the main DOC facility fifty miles away.

* * *

Inside, Hank looks out longingly through the bars at the warm morning sun on the fields outside.

For a moment the mirage returns, and he sees himself easing off the gas going through the fateful turn, waving to the hidden policeman as he drives by.

The bus hits a pothole, forcing the electronic monitor he is sitting on further up his asshole. The mirage shatters with the plug's sudden thrusting penetration, dissolves, leaving in its place a very frightened young man, his stomach knotted. Tensing on the unwanted intruder, waiting in fear for what he knows is coming.

The bus clatters down the road, appearing to hit ever bump and rut in the pavement as it dwindles into a dusty spot of indistinct metal and exhaust fumes... and then is gone ...

❋ ❋ ❋

Half an hour later the bus is stopped again, this time at the end of a dirt driveway that leads up to a dilapidated shack, cracked siding and rusting cars across the lawn. All signs of a distinctly masculine hand. In the windows, tattered curtains, and Hank sees an indistinct face behind them, peering out. A young man's face, about his age.

Hank sits silently in his seat, watching dully as the driver and nurse talk in low voices about ten yards from the front door. From their behavior they appear to be expecting trouble.

Through the open bus window and his own fog of dread, Hank hears snippets of the conversation drifting in on the gentle morning zephyrs. "Repeat offender," he hears the driver say, and sees the man shaking his head as he says it. "Flight risk..." the nurse interjects a few minutes later. And the conversation goes on, but the winds have changed, and now Hank sees the lips of the two men moving off in the distance without hearing their voices. Hank lowers his head, closes his eyes and tenses his rectum against the uncomfortable intruder impaling him there. He dares not look at his seatmates to see if their suffering parallels his.

He does not need to, really. From the faint groans he hears around him, he knows that they too are in distress. The six on the bus sit, immobile, skewered, six plugged asses on six benches in the locked impound section of the bus. Six heads hanging down as the driver and the nurse silently move in on the house, slowly at first, then quickly rushing up towards the porch where the curtains are still waving, the white young face suddenly gone from behind them.

* * *

They capture the terrified man at the back of the house as he stumbles through the rough grass towards the thick woods. Hank hears the commotion and the man's screams and curses but keeps his eyes tightly closed as the sounds grow nearer and he senses the three of them approaching the bus, two walking, the third being dragged.

Hank keeps his eyes closed as he hears the driver reaching up into the cab of the bus and hitting the button to the door, keeps his eyes tightly shut as the door to the rear section of the bus grinds open again, willing himself not even to *imagine*, much less see, what the driver and the nurse are doing.

He hears the sound of something heavy being lifted down from the bus, remembers a large metal folding chair he saw as he climbed the steps.

He hears the chair being opened, hears the heavy thump of someone sitting down on it. Hears the curses and the heavy panting of the young man struggling, recalls the thick arms of the nurse and knows that the man's resistance is futile.

* * *

There is a sudden *bang bang bang* on the side of the bus and Hank jerks erect, his eyes flying open.

Out the window and below him he sees the nurse sitting comfortably on the opened chair, the young man on his stomach over the older man's lap. Struggling in vain against the nurse's thick arm pinning his down, against the worn brown leather wrist and ankle ties that secure his arms and legs. He sees the driver holding a thick leather strap, raising it to hit the bus again, and hears the man yelling to the passengers inside. "You in the bus," the driver bellows, "watch this! So you know what happens to boys who try to escape." The driver hits the bus with the strap again, three loud explosive impacts of heavy saddle leather on its thin metal skin, and the bus shakes and rattles from the impacts, startling the other passengers to quaking attention.

Six frightened faces look down through six barred windows as the driver pulls a large plastic box from the bus, sets it down by the nurse and opens it, slowly, deliberately.

Six frightened faces watch as the driver reaches in and withdraws a large bulb syringe, blue bulb and thick plastic nozzle, fills it from a clear bottle of red viscous fluid.

Six faces watch in fear as the driver opens a jar of Vaseline and plunges the nozzle into the greasy lubricant, hands it to the nurse, who has already stripped the culprit over his knees bare from the waist down, exposing the hairy buttocks, the tightened asscrack, and the dangling genitalia beneath.

The men in the bus watch in terror as the nurse roughly pushes the nozzle up between the ass-cheeks, watches the man over his lap tensing his cheeks together in a futile attempt to stop the entry of the nozzle, crossing his legs in an attempt to deny it admission.

Six bottoms tense in unison as the nurse gives the bulb of the syringe a hard squeeze, tense as the man over the nurse's lap moans and struggles as the liquid is injected into his bowels. Six bottoms tense as the liquid squirts in and stay tensed as the nurse holds the nozzle in place for a long minute after all the liquid has entered.

The nozzle comes out, and the nurse holds it up for inspection. It is not clean. The nurse shakes his head from side to side, says something to the driver, who makes a note on his clipboard.

Now the driver kneels down and retrieves a monitor from the box beside him, hands it to the nurse. The nurse inserts the monitor into the now slack opening of the rectum of the young man across his knees. The man lies over the nurse's lap, spent, unresisting. Or is it the effects of the fluid, the tranquilizer already acting? The monitor is in now, and Hank sees the driver approach, raising the leather strap. Hank screws his eyes shut.

The sounds of the strap striking muscular male buttocks ring out through the early morning, echo off the sides of the bus, off the walls of the shack and down the dirt driveway to the main road. To the ears of passing truck drivers on their way to work. Hank hears the strapping and thinks about his own sentence, hears the man crying and the driver's unmerciful application of the leather to his behind. He opens his eyes when he hears footsteps on the stairs at the end of the bus, sees the man climbing up, head down, sees him turn to sit, his pants still at his knees.

Hank sees the man's angry red cheeks, the strap marks emblazoned across them, and the head of the monitor protruding from in between. The man sits down on the seat across from Hank, gingerly, sideways to favor his blistered ass. He hangs his head, his moans quiet but continuous.

The driver stows the box and the chair, closes the door to the locked section of the bus. He climbs into his seat, the nurse next to him, and starts the motor.

* * *

The bus reverses down the dirt path and back out onto the highway. South again, the DOC facility less than 10 minutes away over the green hills, bright in the morning sun.

Despite the warmth of the day, Hank shivers, thinking about what lies in store for him.

As the bus bounces down the road, the moans of the man across the aisle from Hank increase.

Hank's misery has only just begun.

THE PUNISHMENT

The woman sits alone, behind her desk, facing the room, the windows directly in front of her, the door to the far left. Her clock ticks away in the corner; then, there's a whir as the mechanism moves, the sound of the chimes, soft and sonorous, and, as the reverberations die away, the room once more becomes still.

For a moment that silence holds, the late afternoon sun streaming in through the opening in the curtains, catching the dust motes dancing. Falling across the thick carpeting, across the heavy wooden stool incongruously positioned in the middle of the room, directly in front of the desk, partially obscuring the view of the windows.

The stool: the old dark wood, and the heavy platform that forms its base. Dark wood: so dark that only careful scrutiny reveals the fine scratches along the two front legs, the ones facing away from the desk where the middle-aged woman sits, the ones facing away from the desk and towards the windows.

Scratches: you'll have to look closely to see them, bending close to see the thin parallel lines where fingernails have clawed along the wood; bending close to see where hands have tightened in pain and gripped, dug deep, raked downwards.

The woman sits at her desk, the stool in front of her as yet unoccupied.

There's a heavy wooden paddle to her right, and, beside it, an opened jar of Vaseline. The woman studies the paper on her desk, picks up her pen, and begins to write.

As she writes there's a sound from outside the room, a faint scuffling, as of dragging feet, or perhaps of feet being dragged. A pause, and then a knock. Timid, and the woman at the desk ignores it, although her pen pauses long enough above the page to make it plain that she isn't deaf to the sound, but instead indifferent.

Again the knock, louder, and the woman at the desk places her pen on the paper before her, leans back in her chair. "Enter," she says, and watches as the doorknob turns, and the door opens.

In walks a pretty girl in her middle twenties, head down, her gait slow, reluctant. The door closes loudly behind her.

The girl jumps, upset by the noise. She stands for a moment, her hands trembling.

And then, having calmed herself, she slowly crosses the space between the door and the desk, walking with such hesitation that the older woman waiting finds herself clearing her throat in irritation.

"You know why you're here," she says. "And you know what's coming." The girl's head raises and lowers, barely perceptible, but enough to signify her understanding.

"Lift up your skirt, and bend down over the stool," the woman says.

She doesn't bother to look up to see if she's being obeyed.

＊ ＊ ＊

Hearing the command, the girl turns, drags her feet across to the stool and stops in front of it, her back to the woman at the desk. Slowly the hands reach down behind, finding the fabric of the white skirt that covers the posterior. The skirt rises, exposing the stockinged legs, the upper thighs, and, finally, the firm buttocks presented inside a pair of excessively tight and very sheer underpants.

The girl stands, subdued, waiting. Watching, it's impossible to avoid the feeling that she's been instructed to disrobe in this manner, a sensuous stripping, a slow revealing of her behind in the manner of a carefully choreographed ritual. The ritual of correction.

A pause, as the girl collects herself, and then moves forward to the stool. Bending herself down, she rests her tummy on the seat. The hands release the skirt and move to grip the legs where other hands have gripped before.

In this position, bent tightly over the stool, the bottom is clearly visible through the seat of the underpants. Two twin tightening orbs, and the deep dusky divide between. The cheeks tense and loosen as the girl bends.

After a few minutes, the woman at the desk looks up. For a second or two her eyes take in the scene, the nervous tensing of the raised cheeks, the hands tightly gripping the legs of the stool. Then, having confirmed that the girl is in the instructed position, the woman returns to her writing, at which she labors without pause. Labors without another look at the posterior presented before her.

More time passes. The clock rings in the quarter hour. The underpants of the girl over the stool become damp with perspiration. They cling tighter to the behind, affording a better view of every aspect of the girl's rear anatomy. The thickly folded flesh between the legs, the tight little virginal hole between the cheeks.

The clock rings in the half hour. Then — and only then — does the woman at the desk put her pen down. The girl over the stool hears the sound and tenses. The woman stretches, slowly moves the chair back. Gets up. Pauses, just for a moment, and then approaches her waiting victim.

The middle-aged hand descends, comes to rest on the broadened seat of the underpants. The fingers move across the tightly stretched fabric, teasing the firm young flesh beneath. No noise in the room other than the faint whisper of flesh brushing silk, and the labored breathing of the girl over the stool.

For a long moment the older woman fondles the buttocks, letting her hand run across them, the broad expanse in the center, the tapering thighs below.

For a long moment the older woman fondles the buttocks, an aperitif of sorts, an appetizer for the events that are about to unfold.

For the discipline that is about to begin.

※　※　※

She's been doing this for longer than she can remember, so long that her actions have become second nature. The positioning, the examination that precedes correction. She no longer stops to think about what she's doing, about the effects of her actions on the culprit.

That there is an effect is undeniable; the hand on the seat of the underpants, the proprietary handling, they cannot fail but have an effect. Alone in the room with her chastiser, the girl waits, her behind lifted, her cheeks slightly separated by her positioning over the stool. Her face is bent down so that she cannot see what is happening to her backside, but the combination of the noises that she hears and attempts to interpret, the hand on her buttocks, emphasizing the girl's own lack of control and lack of privacy, and the images running wild in her mind all combine to evoke both fear and a peculiar sense of calm.

The hand moves across the girl's behind, proprietary, saying — without words — "this is not yours to control, it is mine, and mine alone." The older woman does it naturally, smoothing the cool fabric over the taught cheeks, stopping to adjust the underpants so that they sit perfectly over the smooth round contours of the young bottom that waits for the punishment.

The hand smooths the fabric, first over the center of the buttocks, and then down between them, pressing in firmly in the crevasse between, tickling the anus through the thin cloth, raising the prospect of its punishment in the mind of the girl over the stool. The girl, still a virgin in that area, tenses against the finger. The hand raises, descends on the buttocks with a sharp smack. A warning of the penalty for failure to cooperate. The finger is reintroduced to the tight anus, deeper this time.

Now, despite the increased humiliation of the penetration, the cheeks do not tense. Instead, the girl struggles to be still and to keep herself presented, over the stool, her behind high in the air.

As she feels the finger move, pushing in as far as the fabric will allow, her stomach tightens at the realization that her chastiser will not allow the fabric to interfere with the punishment.

And that, therefore, the descent of the knickers is only moments away.

❈　❈　❈

The older woman begins to lecture, scolding the culprit as she withdraws her finger, drags it slowly up the crack, the onslaught against the prim little anus diminishing as the finger moves. Up it goes, towards the waistband of the panties. The hand rests there for a minute, the voice scolding now, rising in volume as each point is made.

The fingers slip inside the panties, go back down. The intrusion into the anus resumes, this time without the thin fabric of the panties to interfere, this time without any allowance for the culprit's modesty, or inexperience in that area.

The tip of the finger presses firmly against the entrance to the tight button. The voice becomes harsher. The free hand rises to grip firmly between the spread legs, pushing down into the sex between them. Manualizing the culprit as the lecture continues.

Imagine the scene: the young woman, prone over the stool, skirt raised, buttocks upthrust, covered only by the thin film of the panties; the older woman standing behind, one hand down the panties with a thin finger penetrating the anus, the other masturbating the girl between her legs as she bends, waiting.

At first there will be a sharp intake of breath at the intrusion of the hand. And then, resistance will set in, and the girl will attempt to retain her dignity by refusing to respond to the stimulation. The older woman will notice the locked legs, the tightened buttocks, and will rub harder in response.

As she does so the culprit will begin to react. A slight movement at first, an almost imperceptible rocking motion. More obvious is the tightening of the anus, involuntary, but noticeable, particularly as it occurs in synchrony with the motions of the hand between the legs.

In response, the older woman's finger will move further into the bottom, teasing, the finger deeper into the anus at the same time that the fingers in between the legs withdraw. A rhythm ensues, one finger moving in while the other retreats, and then the original finger withdrawing while the retracted finger is reinserted. The culprit responds, despite herself, finds herself moving backward and forward to maximize her pleasure, finds herself responding to the stimulation the older woman provides. Responding despite herself.

The odor of arousal fills the room. The girl begins to moan, the rocking grows more noticeable.

The fingers move more vigorously now, thrusting in and out of the pussy and anus. The panties are still up, hindering the motion of the finger in the bottom, but in some odd way their presence adds to the excitement the girl over the stool feels. Fear-induced, in all likelihood; fear, from the knowledge that her humiliation is only partial, that she is already stripped of her modesty without being stripped of all her clothes.

Her excitement grows at that thought, a part of her mind conjuring an image of herself bent over — panties lowered — and the humiliation of that position, the humiliation of being masturbated, of having her behind penetrated and her sex stimulated.

Her excitement grows, and she feels the tingling growing inside her. The older woman appears oblivious; the fingers continue their motions despite the moans, despite the obvious arousal.

Closer and closer the culprit comes, until she feels herself hovering on the edge, on the brink of orgasm, about to achieve release.

The older woman's timing is, as always, impeccable. Just as the girl feels herself ready, the rubbing stops.

The finger against the clitoris withdraws. As does the finger in the behind.

In just a few seconds, bliss ends, fear sets in.

Fear, as the hands quickly slide into the panties, yank them down.

Fear, as the fog of the arousal dissipates, and the culprit recalls the jar of Vaseline on the table.

And the heavy wooden paddle.

＊　＊　＊

The older woman crosses to her desk, leaving the culprit bent over the stool, her ardor dissipated, the presence of the fingers in front and in back a memory.

The girl over the stool cannot see what is happening behind her, but she hears noises that make her tummy churn. The sound of the paddle being moved across the surface of the desk; the sound of the drawer being opened, and of something being withdrawn. A sharp metallic sound, metal against the wood of the desktop — and then all is quiet.

The girl hangs over the stool, still feeling the teasing intrusion of the fingers in her pussy, and in her behind. Once again she finds herself envisioning the scene, the bottom — her bottom — bared and stuck up, everything displayed, nothing hidden from view.

The sound of footsteps behind her, coming closer… closer… and then suddenly turning away as the older woman heads to the door to her office. The girl hears the door open, the footsteps diminishing outside, going down the corridor. A muffled thud of another door being opened, and the girl recalls the bathroom she had seen earlier. The faint sound of water running in the taps confirms her suspicion.

The girl waits there for the water to be shut off, for the footsteps to grow louder, for the older woman to return.

✻　✻　✻

Anticipation is, of course, a fundamental part of the discipline; it builds the mood, allows the culprit awaiting chastisement to conjure her own worst nightmares. So the older woman ensures that there is a long delay while the girl waits, bent over the stool. Ensures that she provides enough suggestions to set the girl's imagination wild.

Suggestions: the sight of the paddle, and of the Vaseline. The lubricant intended for one purpose, the preparation of the behind for penetration. The girl knows this — has heard the stories — but, even knowing, the sight of the jar there on the desk is disconcerting. Discomfiting. The rendering real of that which, until this moment, has been nothing more than a fear pushed to the dark recesses of her mind.

Suggestions: the punishment room, the mere repetition of the words enough to cause a shiver down the spine. The girl has heard of it; has walked past the corridor that leads to it; has even imagined what its interior might hold; but, until this moment, has never entered it. Now, from the moment she crossed the threshold, its reality presses down on her, an oppressive weight that only a major distraction can lift. A major distraction, such as the one afforded by the older woman's hand between the girl's legs, and a finger up the behind.

Suggestions: the stool, and the scratches on the legs that indicate to the girl that she is not the first to be bent over it, not the first to feel the humiliation of having to stick her behind up for the attentions to it that the older woman chooses to inflict.

Suggestions: the wait over the stool, unable to see what is happening behind her, having to rely instead on sounds and scents. Bent over, alone in the room, bared bottom facing the opened door, aware of how revealed she is, the girl waits, listening for footsteps.

Which, finally, she hears, returning from the bathroom, growing louder in the hallway, coming into the room.

The door closes. The footsteps go to the desk, pause, and then come slowly towards the stool.

The older woman comes into view. In her hands she carries a large tray. On it, a large bar of soap, cut into quarters and sitting in a deep bowl; a two-quart pitcher of water; and, finally a medium-sized hand towel, rising in a low mound over an indeterminate object underneath it.

The woman sets the tray down on the floor in front of the culprit, goes to the desk, and returns with her chair. She sits down on it, reaches down and lifts the pitcher. Carefully, she pours water from it onto the cut pieces of soap, enough water to just reach the top of each piece.

She sets the pitcher down, pauses for a moment. Then she reaches down and picks up two pieces of soap, one by one, each already partially dissolved from sitting in the water. Holding her hand over the pitcher, she methodically squeezes each piece through her fingers, watching the soft soap oozing out and then dropping down into the pitcher.

The water inside turns cloudy. The woman picks up the third piece of soap, holds it in both hands, and rolls it slowly between them. The soap deforms into a long cylinder. The woman continues to roll until the cylinder is smooth. Satisfied, she sets it aside.

She now turns her attention to the remaining soap quarter. For the first time she looks directly into the girl's eyes, reaching her hand out to hold her chin, tilting her head so that she can be sure of her audience.

Holding the head with one hand, she reaches the other down to the remaining quarter of soap. She picks it up, holding it for a moment over the bowl, letting the excess liquid drip down.

"Open your mouth," she says. The girl hesitates. The woman's free hand comes up quickly, taps the girl across her right cheek, not hard, but with enough force to turn the head slightly to one side.

"Open your mouth," the woman says, this time more softly, almost inviting rather than commanding. A pause, and then the lips move, the mouth opens.

The older woman slips the quarter piece of soap in, gently pushes up on the lower jaw with her free hand.

She stands. Strokes the back of the girl's head, the back of the neck, then leans down and removes the towel from the tray, which she uses to wipe the hand that held the soap.

She becomes aware of a change in the breathing pattern of the culprit. She looks down.

There before both of them sits the tray. With the towel removed, the apparatus of correction previously hidden by it are now completely visible.

The metal syringe, a squat shiny chromed barrel, and a tapering metal nozzle. The plunger pulled back, indicating that it has already been primed with fluid, primed for introduction and administration into the waiting backside.

The metal syringe, ready to be used. And: a latex enema bag, empty, and a very large plastic nozzle at the end of the hose.

The utility of the pitcher of water — now very soapy — is all too clear.

The culprit groans. Suggestion has given way to reality.

A conclusion that becomes inescapable as the woman reaches, picks up the metal syringe, and walks out of sight behind the waiting girl.

A long pause. Standing in front of the girl, her bent figure blocking the actions of the woman behind her, the sharp intake of breath and the sudden tightening of the girl's hands on the legs of the stool are the only indicators that the cold metal nozzle had been inserted into the behind.

A faint sound from behind her, and the hands grip tighter still. The bottom sways slightly from side to side and, inside the shoes, the toes are no doubt curled.

All evidence that the woman is squeezing the plunger, and that the injection of fluid into her virgin bowels, has begun.

❋ ❋ ❋

She is unable to decide which is more effective, enemas given with the syringe, or enemas administered using the two-quart bag hanging above the culprit's head. The syringe has the advantage of being convenient: the scolding; the taking down of the panties; the trip over the knee; the insertion and injection of the contents of the syringe; cornertime with the bared bottom on display, waiting until the culprit does the potty dance; and, finally, the release, either alone or, if greater humiliation is desired, in front of the older woman.

On the other hand, the syringe is unsuitable for the delivery of large volume, which in turn is desirable for the strong need for expulsion it induces. True, the syringe can be removed, refilled, and reinserted, with enough such cycles resulting in the net administration of a considerable amount of solution. And the effect of the repeated penetration of the culprit's behind with the syringe's nozzle is salutary.

But the gradual introduction of the solution into the recipient's bottom is often too soothing. What is required for most of her charges is the short sharp shock. The sudden surging of the solution down the tube, through the nozzle, past the anus and into the depths of the bowels. The unrelenting flow, and the helplessness that comes from that sudden and continuous introduction of fluid. Knowing the daunting size of the bag, knowing the pressure will continue to mount and mount and mount — and the only respite is that afforded by the older woman's decision to close the clamp. Whether for an instant or an hour, up to her and to her alone.

And then of course there is also the psychological to be considered. The syringe is threatening, but the bag is daunting. It hangs there, in front of the culprit for her to look at, swaying slightly, the hose hanging, the nozzle already Vaselined. When she's had to deal with two or three girls at once she's found it particularly effective to have all three bags hanging in her office; she can still recall the exact expression on each face, wondering which will be for her, especially if she chooses to fill one considerably more than the others. She can also recall the sight of three red behinds standing side by side against the wall across from her desk; three red bottoms, a long rubber hose dangling from each, and three pairs of feet shifting uncomfortably as three sets of bowels cried out desperately for relief.

The image fades as she returns her attention to the girl in front of her. All the solution that the syringe contained is now in the tensing bowels, and so she withdraws the nozzle, watching carefully as she pulls it clear, making sure that the puckered opening grips it tightly.

"No leakage," she had said as she first inserted the nozzle. The tone was calm, conversational really, as if she were discussing the weather at afternoon tea. But of course the girl knew the threat that lay behind the words; and the older woman is pleased to see that the anus squeezes tight as the nozzle is withdrawn, the girl tensing in order to ensure that everything inside her remains inside.

The nozzle comes completely clear of the behind, and the woman walks in front of the girl and puts the syringe down on the tray.

"We'll hold that a bit while we think about what we've done," she says, this time adopting a lilting tone, as if speaking to a child still in nappies. "We'll hold that a bit, and then we'll have the full bag as punishment for our ghastly behavior."

She reaches back down to the tray, retrieves the quarter of soap that she has shaped into a cylinder, walks back behind the girl.

"But from your actions I imagine you are not the kind of girl who can be trusted to achieve the task set for you without some assistance," she says, speaking to the back of the girl's head; aware that the drooping down of that head indicates the mortification of the culprit at the words she hears.

"And so I've decided to aid you in your obedience. So be a good girl now and push your bottom back for me. And remember, this is for your own good. Since, after all, if you were to leak I'd have to cane you. And you wouldn't want that, now would you?"

As she talks one hand reaches out and spreads the cheeks, the other places the head of the soap cylinder against the tight orifice. Slowly it is inserted, the white soap disappearing as it ascends into the already filled bowels.

When the entire cylinder is inside, the woman walks to the other side of the stool, reaches down and holds her hand underneath the girl's mouth.

"Let it out now," she says, gently. The jaw drops, the remnants of the piece of soap fall into the older woman's hand. She puts them in the tray, picks the towel up and wipes the residue of soap off the mouth.

She puts the towel down, pats the girl's cheek, strokes her hair for a moment — and then returns to her desk.

Sitting there, she looks down at her work; then, she looks up at the girl.

She smiles. "After you've had the enema in your bottom for a while, I'm going to fill the bag and put the nozzle in, and give you all of its contents too."

She puts a hand down between her legs, moving it there slowly so that her lover can see her doing it.

"And then, since it was your idea, I'm going to make you hold the enema while I fuck your bottom with the phallus you bought me."

Her lover, of course, has nothing to say. Partially because the residual soap in her mouth makes speaking difficult.

But mostly because she has no need to say anything.

The evening is perfect enough already.

Why ruin it with words?

After all, words ruin everything.

TWELVE STEPS TO EFFECTIVE ANTICIPATION

Note: These Twelve Steps have been written for a recipient of the female gender. However, the reader will have little difficulty adapting them to a male recipient if desired.

1. *Whenever possible, the recipient should be informed of the approach of the procedure well in advance, allowing for time to come to terms with its inevitability as well as to purchase the clothes to be worn during the preparation and for the ceremony itself. A more visceral reminder of the preparation and ceremony is often appropriate.*

She stands at her closet later on in the morning, after she's come back from shopping. Staring with great difficulty at the two feet of space she's cleared, and at what's hanging there for her to view every morning when she dresses, every evening when she changes before bed.

The trip itself wasn't difficult, she reflects, at least not in comparison to the anxiety she felt coming to terms with the fact of her going. The *necessity* of her going. Once she had made the decision, it was easy to go to her closet to select the clothes she would wear, white puerile panties, shorts, and a blouse.

And so she dressed, walked down to the car and got in. Drove to the mall. Not the closest, but one a good distance away, feeling her tension rising as the miles rolled by under the wheels and she felt the tight fabric of her panties against her bottom cheeks. Felt the wetness between her legs. She drove to the mall and walked slowly from her parked car to the lingerie store, feeling the eyes of the clerks on her as she shopped there, the lone customer. Walking slowly around the store, selecting the things she's imagined wearing, her imagination conjuring the images for her as she lay in bed the night before, unable to sleep. The images in bed, and their partial confirmation as she stood before the full-length mirror that morning.

She stood before the mirror wearing a white blouse and thin cotton panties, and thought about wearing a skirt. Pleated perhaps, like a schoolgirl... or just black and thin and short. She turned to face her seat towards the mirror and, looking back over her shoulder, bent over slowly, awkwardly, feeling herself blush as she watched the hem of her blouse lifting up over the tight twin cheeks of her behind. Watched the hem rise like a curtain on a stage, imagined it was the hem of her skirt rising instead. Imagined the seat of her panties coming slowly into view. "The target," she could not stop herself from thinking.

Ultimately she bought both skirts, the pleated one, the thin black one. Carried them with her into the changing room along with the panties she had imagined. Changed, and stood in front of the mirror in the little room, bending over, looking back. Watching in fascination and fear as the hem rose, revealing her thighs, the lower curves of her cheeks and, finally, the white seat of the panties, sheer in back, the two white moons beneath clearly visible, as well as the dark vertical crack between them. She wondered what she would look like bending with a plug in her behind, the pink base of the plug visible underneath her panties, a reminder to her and to any observer of the events that were about to take place.

She held her pose for a long moment, twisting her head back to the mirror to observe herself, seeing herself as she knew she would be seen. Seeing her skirt up in back and her cheeks white beneath her panties. Feeling the eyes she knew would be on her, already anticipating the sensation of her panties being lowered, hearing the sharp command ringing out in the air, shuffling her legs further apart as she reaches her hands back to obey.

To withdraw the rectal plug, the reminder of preparation and ceremony.

To put a hand on each cheek to separate them.

To feel the Vaselined nozzle being inserted.

She stands at her closet, looking at the skirts and panties that she's hung there, thinking about their use in the ritual she knows she's going to experience.

---

2.   *It is also appropriate to have the recipient purchase some of the items used for the preparation and for the ceremony. The recipient should be informed, however, that what occurs will not be under her control, and that there will be equipment available for use that is more exotic and appropriate than any of the basic items she has been instructed to obtain.*

She's changed now, wearing the pleated skirt and panties, and sits on her bed staring at the shopping bag she's brought back from the drugstore. Staring, not yet daring to touch it. Not daring to open it to view its contents, not yet. It doesn't matter, of course, because she knows what's inside, remembers each item in vivid detail.

She remembers walking in the drugstore, wearing her new clothing, feeling the cold air on her bare legs, the swooshing of the skirt as she walks towards the pharmacy, looking for the right aisle. She finds it, feeling butterflies in her tummy as she walks its length, trying not to look obvious; feeling naked there, feeling her cheeks flush and eyes on her back. She walks the length of the aisle, slowly, too nervous to stop, reaching its end and turning the corner, the contents of the aisle still vivid in her mind.

She waits a long moment, catching her breath, and then turns and walks back, walks down the aisle to the section she's just left.

She takes them in order, the order in which she imagines they will be used, gingerly lifting each object down to her basket as if it might burn her. The thermometer first, and the large jar of Vaseline with it. She reads the packages carefully, looks past the oral thermometers, finds the baby ones, her eyes passing smoothly over the word "Baby" without pause, some force inside her driving her to look until the synonym slips into view: "Rectal." "Rectal thermometer," the words she dares not speak, but even moving her lips voicelessly over the syllables she shivers. She lowers the rectal thermometer from the shelf to her basket, adds the jar of Vaseline, moves on down the aisle.

In her head a sort of juvenile grammar springs into her mind. Vaseline. To Vaseline. To be Vaselined. She is Vaselined. She is going to be Vaselined. She waits to be Vaselined, for the Vaseline, for him to Vaseline her.

"She is waiting to have her panties pulled down to feel him Vaselining her," she thinks, coming to a halt before the Fleet enemas.

She silently adds a Fleet to her basket, followed by a jar of glycerin suppositories. The enema bag is last, a combination hot water bottle, douche bag, enema bag. She pauses for a moment. Adds the box to her basket.

She pays a male clerk, blushing furiously red as he scrutinizes her and her purchases. She is dripping when she finally escapes from the store; as she leaves she is left with the sense of the clerk's eyes staring at her, staring at her behind underneath her short skirt.

She hurries to the safety of her car and the ride back home.

She is uncomfortably aware of the pressure of the seat against her bottom. And the shopping bag next to her.

---

3.   *In order to encourage meditations upon the upcoming preparation and ceremony, the recipient should be required to write lines or by some other means convey an understanding of what is expected of her, as well as of what she herself expects will occur.*

She's laid her purchases out in front of her on her desk, and sits now, writing.

Before writing, she's taken off her skirt and panties. Standing in front of her mirror, she's undressed, imagining having to do this on Friday. Allowing herself to feel some of the fear and anticipation she knows she'll feel when the time comes.

She writes:

I'm sitting at my desk, writing this letter in order to work through in my own mind the feelings I'm having. I've had several days to think about it, and even if I had tried to put

what's going to occur out of my mind, I find that these emotions are too powerful to deny.

It surprises me to say that. Two days ago if someone had told me that I would feel this excitement I would have laughed. I would have responded that I felt distaste, perhaps even a bit of curiosity, but certainly not excitement.

So why is it that I'm feeling that now... excitement? Excitement, anticipation, fear. All of that... why am I feeling it?

I think part of the answer is in the sequence of events that I've experienced. There's a physical part to this – an undeniable physical part – but so much more of it is mental. If someone had just taken me into a room and done it, I think my reaction would have been completely different. But doing it this way, telling me in advance, exposing me to it every day, an escalation of exposure, it's had an effect on me.

It's so... deliberate. And deliberative. I feel as if everything is planned, including my own reactions. My own thoughts, the way my body feels... is that under my control or yours? How can you know me better than I know myself? Play my body and my mind, turn me into the instrument of your desires?

When I was first told, I felt mostly fear. But now I feel such excitement too, and I feel as if I've been marched there, fed forbidden fruits, slowly, morsel by morsel, so that everything has been under my control and *nothing* has been under my control. How can that be? Both at the same time?

In the course of only a few days I've been... brainwashed? Overwhelmed by what I've seen and heard? If I had only read about what I've already done today – would I feel the same?

All I've been able to do today is to think about what I've already learned, and to think about what's coming next. My body has a will of its own, my mind has locked onto a goal that it will attain. How can all of this happen without any command, without any physical presence? What is there inside me that allows this to happen? Is this something I want?

It must be. It's all so real to me; even though I haven't had it yet I've played it through in my mind so often that I feel as if I've done it once, twice, many times. I'm in my room waiting for you, lying on my bed, on my tummy, with my panties down. I imagine you coming for me.

I imagine hearing you coming up the stairs, walking down the hallway towards me. When I was a child my mom kept the medicines in the hall closet, above our reach, and that's where I imagine you keeping the bag. I imagine you stopping there, and me hearing your footsteps stopping and then the sound of the closet door opening, and I get chills knowing what you're doing. In my mind I see you reaching up to the top shelf and getting out the cardboard box you keep there and carrying it down the hall towards me. I know what's in the box and my bottomhole is already tensing at the thought of it. I'm excited and scared lying there waiting, and I know if I checked myself now I would be very, very wet. Is that wrong?

I can't stop thinking about this. I imagine you coming into my room with the box and some other things, and you looking at me and telling me that you're unhappy with me and that we have some things to attend to. You don't say it yet, but I know that you're going to tell me that I've been naughty and that I deserve to have the naughtiness washed out of me. I think about needing to have a washout, and I imagine your making me say that, a "washout." Or, worse, having to write it before you do it, sitting bare-bottomed at my desk the way I am now, writing, over and over, "I have been a naughty girl and so I deserve the spanking and punishment enema Daddy is about to give me."

I never thought I would want to call anyone daddy, but I feel the power of the word, and it makes me feel good to say it. What I've thought about isn't incestuous, it's... loving. I like that. It excites me.

I imagine it all starting when you come out of my bathroom, and of watching as you sit down on a chair and gesture to me to come to you. I'm over your lap with you pulling down my panties as you scold me, and I know that it's the last time my bottom will be white for several days. I tense my cheeks when you put your hand on them, but realize you are only laying it there while you lecture; this intimacy makes me feel loved and embarrasses me even more because I know in a minute you'll be spanking me.

And you do, but first you make me watch in a mirror as you get out the rectal thermometer and shake it down and put Vaseline on it. "That naughty girl in the mirror is having her temperature taken the old-fashioned way," I think to myself, "over her Daddy's lap with her panties down with a rectal thermometer." I am able to dissociate like that until I feel you pulling my cheeks apart and the tickling sensation of the cold thermometer sliding into me.

I know at this point I will want to close my eyes but I know you won't let me, that you'll want me to see myself in the mirror, bare-bottomed over your lap with the thermometer sticking out. When I was little I remember being at a friend's house and seeing her get her temperature taken that way; she had been sick but had gotten well enough to play but her mom came in during our tea party and told her she needed to check. I remember being fascinated as she pulled down my friend's panties and put her over her lap and I remember looking at my friend's unhappy face and at the thin little thermometer in her behind. I think about you taking my temperature that way, or of who else you might have do it... would there be a nurse? Would I have it done with some other people watching?

After the temperature you spank me, and I feel myself getting sore as the smacks descend. There's a physical sensation I know, a spanking leaves you sore, but there's also the embarrassment of it, of being over someone's lap bare-bottomed. When I think about it I imagine myself wearing something sexier, garters and stockings, and I imagine the pain and the squirming I'll do. But mostly I imagine how I will feel with you in control and me over your lap, head-down, bottom-up. I'm not submissive, not in the sense of just saying fine to anything, but I know that by the end of the spanking I will be eager to please. Is that strange?

And after the spankings, the enemas. I know so much about that part now, and yet I know so little. I knew what I was getting in the store today; I have an idea in my mind of what will happen to me. I imagine you sending me to stand in the corner after you've spanked me and I imagine you telling me that I've been very naughty and that I'm going to get a thorough washout because of that.

And then you tell me that a thorough washout is to clean me out for two reasons. The first is to wash the naughtiness out of me, to make me think about the consequences of misbehavior. And the second reason… I feel my cheeks clench when you tell me that the second reason is that I'm being thoroughly washed out as preparation, that I'm going to get a bottoms-up-cheeks-apart after I'm cleaned. And I know what that means, it means a long session of disciplinary anal sex while I'm bent over the Sodomy Stool. I know you will be very careful in how you do it, that you'll use a condom and be gentle, and that the discipline is really mostly mental and not physical. And it excites me and scares me to know I'll be getting it.

And I stand in the corner and wait for the enemas. I know you'll use a Fleet first, and that I'll be over your lap for it, a juvenile posture for it, having to reach back and hold my own cheeks apart to feel the tickling again as you slide the little nozzle in. I know you'll look down and enjoy that sight, me over your lap with the bottle pressed deep between my cheeks, and I know I'll tense up as you squeeze the bottle and I feel the solution going in. What I don't know is how long you'll keep me there to hold it, or whether you'll put a rectal plug in to help me retain. And if you do, whether you'll send me to stand in the corner with my bare red bottom and the base of the plug on display.

Even though I've never had one I know you'll use a Fleet first to get me ready for the bag enema, and while I retain the Fleet I'll hear you filling the bag in the bathroom, preparing a soapsuds enema. I remember talking to a friend about the enema she got in the hospital – she cried when the male nurse came in with the bag and hung it by her bed, she pleaded with him not to do it but really neither one of them had a choice. And, she told me, soon it was time and the bag was hanging bulging from the IV stand over her head and the nurse was asking her to turn on her side. And she felt him raising up the top flap of the hospital gown she had had to put on, and she felt him lifting one of her cheeks and using his gloved finger to lubricate her back there. I don't know what he used or how he did it – I assume KY jelly and a light touch of a fingertip against her back there – but I imagine it being a more deliberate process in my case. I imagine tensing at the soft pressure of the Vaselined finger, tensing, unsuccessfully, against the slow forceful insertion of that finger into my bottom. Tensing while whoever is doing it moves that finger in and out so I'm thoroughly lubricated and still feeling the intrusion of that finger even when it's finally withdrawn.

I don't know if I'll cry the way she did when he put the tube in, if I'll cry when I hear the *click* of the clamp and feel the soapsuds going into my behind. She didn't go into all the details, but I've been able to imagine it, what happened to her. The usual hospital room, two beds, her roommate in the other and hers with a curtain being drawn around it, the nurse drawing the curtain but the bag already hanging and my friend already on her side. The curtain closed now, and behind it she's feeling that loss of control to a man she's never seen before, a complete stranger who is compelling her to show herself to him. To show her bare bottom, to show the intimate orifice between her cheeks. Lying on her side behind that curtain feeling a complete stranger standing there looking down at her, tickling her between her bare cheeks with his finger, in preparation for the insertion of the tube.

I think a lot about that. I wonder what it feels like, how I'll react to it. I think about that and about the sensation of the soapsuds going in. Of lying there under someone else's control feeling myself filling up, slowly. I know I'll trust whoever is doing it… I know they'll use a safe solution, a low pressure, a careful insertion and new equipment. But what will it feel like when it happens?

I guess I'll find out. About the enema, and the expulsion. And the Sodomy Stool which, in my mind, is standing there in the middle of the room. Waiting.

---

4.   *The recipient should be given final written instructions on the morning of the proceedings, and these instructions should be delivered in a way known to the recipient, thereby maximizing the recipient's anticipation of the day's activities. She should be required to acknowledge receipt of these final instructions; writing repeated lines of text is effective here as well.*

---

5.   *Some procedure should be employed to monitor the recipient's state of anticipation throughout the day. Periodic phone calls are particularly effective in this regard.*

---

6.   *The recipient should be instructed in advance on how to prepare for the arrival of the lover, the disciplinarian, the nurse, or whoever it is that will be carrying out the proceedings. Preparation should be deliberate, and should be accompanied by audiovisual aids for the recipient to ponder. It is often appropriate to supply a camera (still or video) or even tape recorder so that the recipient can record her preparations for later review. Such recording must of course be consensual, not covert, and must be shared only by those involved except by agreement.*

She looks at the pictures she's found, at the stories she has collected to read. She's never sure of their reality: are the pictures real or are they clever composites? Are they models with rouged bottoms, or the real recipients of someone's strict ministrations?

These days reality has taken on a different meaning for her. What is the reality behind the words on the screen? Are the stories she reads true, or the products of someone's imagination? Do the pictures lie?

It's not an academic question. She finds herself consumed with thoughts of the upcoming event, and wonders whether she is abnormal for finding it so appealing as well as terrifying. She finds stories written by other women expressing similar emotions, finds sites devoted to what she's about to experience. Is it real? Or is she a freak for having these desires, for wanting to respond to them.

As she reads she realizes that it must be real, most of it. The emotions described are too familiar. She finds one site which strikes her as having been written just for her. As she reads the stories she finds there she realizes that she feels things the story describes the reader as feeling, almost as if someone were looking out through the monitor and into her mind as she read.

As she reads this site she learns – learns not just about what's going to happen to her, but about why she responds to it. The expression of caring that underlies it all, the desire to give up control to someone who will be kind to her. Someone who will take the power and shelter her from the world, if only for a time, if only imperfectly. She realizes it's a regression of sorts, to a childhood lived and lost, or in many cases never lived at all, and sought after ever since.

She looks at the pictures and imagines the women who appear in them, not as models, but as real people, responding to what they experience. This one, undressed from the waist down and bending over a man's lap. What is she feeling? Pain and embarrassment, yes. But are those sensations and emotions bad? Or are they a way of her releasing the things she feels and cannot express? A catharsis of sorts, letting someone else make the decisions for her, judge her, condemn her and carry out the punishment. Helping her to atone for whatever it is she's done – whatever it is she imagines she's done. Catharsis and closure. At the hands of someone decent, someone the woman in the picture respects. Someone who cares.

She looks at the pictures on this site and reads the stories and the letters. She reads about the "Discipline Project," the letters and pictures of women who have agreed to be corrected, to have their correction recorded for others to witness. Why would someone do this? She thinks about atonement, about the confessional booth and, in the early church, the scourging of penitents. She realizes that the act of contrition is a liberating one, and that someone understands that, and the needs that lie behind it.

After all, ceremony has always played an important part of human life. Every tribe has rites of passage, acts that are performed when a boy becomes a man, a girl a woman. When a child is born the community celebrates, and when an adult dies the community grieves. When someone commits a crime the punishment is before the group, a collective judging, a collective purging of sin.

Even when there is no crime, no sin, the individual places herself within the group, punishes herself for her failure, real or perceived. She thinks of Foucault's argument that modern society depends upon the internalization of conformity, that instead of society inflicting punishment on the individual, in the modern world it is the individual herself who seeks to conform, who punishes herself through guilt when she does not. She realizes how true it is, how she feels bad for every act she has promised herself she will perform and doesn't, for every character failing she vows to correct and cannot, for every sin she feels she has committed, no matter how trivial such failings are by any objective criterion.

She looks at the pictures she's found, red bottoms, a girl bent over with a double-bardex inflated, the ones from the "Discipline Project" website. She wonders what it would be like to be purged of guilt, to submit herself to someone else, not out of weakness but out of respect and a desire for catharsis. Knowing she has done wrong, knowing that the slate will be wiped clean.

She reads, and as she reads she realizes that she is not alone. What she wants is simply to be loved. To be protected in whatever approximation of childhood one adult can give another. To be listened to. To be respected. And to have limits set and enforced. Not through anger, but through punishment. Through corporal punishment. Through a loss of control and a loss of dignity. Things no child should experience but that she, as an adult, can consent to.

She spends a long time reading the stories and looking at the pictures trying to understand. At the end, she realizes that she is not alone in how she feels and what she wants.

And this is a great relief to her.

---

7.   *Part of the process of preparation should include practicing the positions that will be employed during the procedures. Although these positions should be rehearsed immediately before the actual events, practice well in advance of these events has been shown to have a salutary effect on the recipient.*

She begins to wonder how it would feel to be positioned like the women she sees in the pictures she has found.

She's already imagined being bent over the bathtub, finds herself looking at the rim of the tub every time she enters the room, imagining how the cold porcelain will feel against her tummy, how she will look bent over with her bottom up in the air. The images in her mind grow stronger, and she finds herself standing in front of the tub as if in a dream, pulling her panties down, looking down at the towel she's put over the rim. She gets down on her knees, slowly, and slides forward over the rim until her head rests against the floor of the tub. She lies there for a very long time, feeling the blood pooling in her head, feeling the cold air blowing across her backside, aware of her vulnerability, of the separation of her cheeks and all that she knows she must be displaying as she holds her pose.

She gets up, goes to her bedroom and gets the bag of purchases from the drugstore. Walks back into the bathroom, her panties still down, and lays the objects out on the counter by the sink. She picks up the thermometer first, tears open the plastic and opens the case. Removing the thermometer slowly, she washes it in cold water from the sink and shakes it down. Imagines looking up from the position she was just in to watch someone else doing it. She puts Vaseline on it and sets it down on the floor near the tub.

She repeats the process with the Fleet and finally the bag, which she assembles standing there with her panties down. Filling it with soapy water from the sink, hanging it from the towel rack. Standing a moment looking at it, how it sways, at the larger douche nozzle which she's chosen to use. At how slick the nozzle is with Vaseline. She lets it hang, goes to her room and comes back with a long mirror, which she props up against the wall opposite the tub.

She could have used a video camera, of course, and thinks to herself that the next time she will. But for now the mirror is enough, and she looks back into it imagining someone else's hand pushing the thermometer into her backside, focusing her attention alternately on the hand pushing it into her bare bottom, and on the sensation of the cold glass inside her. She repeats the process with the tip of the Fleet and then the enema nozzle, spending a long nervous moment looking back at herself with the hose hanging down from between her bare white cheeks. She imagines them red. She finds her hand slipping down between her legs. She rubs, so very aware of the sensation of fullness in her bottom from the slight width of the nozzle. She wonders how much fuller she would feel with the enema inside her.

She knows that all she has to do is to reach up to open the clamp that separates her bottom from the full bag over her head to find out. For the moment she leaves the clamp closed. And rubs.

And thinks about someone else's hand on that clamp. With her waiting there helplessly.

Waiting to hear that *click*.

---

8.   *Immediately before the preparation and ceremony the recipient should be shown the room or rooms where the procedures will be carried out.*

---

9.   *The recipient should also be asked to examine the objects that will be employed. It is advisable to have her arrange them for use, to explain their function.*

---

10. *When all is ready, the recipient should assume the first position, and present herself to the lover, the disciplinarian, the nurse, or whoever it is that will be carrying out the proceedings. She should maintain that position, for as long as is deemed appropriate. Then, and only then, the preparations should begin.*

She wanders through her rooms, the nozzle still in her behind, the hose hanging down, carrying the bag in her hand as she shuffles forward, panties at her knees. She thinks of Diogenes, in search of an honest man, and knows the trait she seeks is somewhat different.

She shuffles through her rooms, and in each she finds herself looking for an appropriate spot. In the kitchen she bends forward over the back of one of the chairs, hanging the bag from the light. In the living room she kneels on the sofa and lifts herself forward so that she is half over its back. The bag hangs down from a side light, and she wonders at the view she presents to the neighbors, for she's left the blinds slightly open.

Through the house she wanders, and in each she finds a favorite spot, a spot where she wants it to happen, if it has to happen at all. Madness perhaps, or perhaps its just her determination to control the circumstances as much as she can. She does not like parties, but when she goes she is determined to be the best-dressed woman there. It's the same thing here, she thinks to herself.

She is methodical, and, within a short period of time has constructed a mental list of spots throughout the house where she might position herself or be positioned. They exist in a hierarchy in her mind; her bedroom is her favorite. So she shuffles back upstairs and moves her full-length mirror to face the bed, hangs the bag from a bedpost. She climbs over some pillows so that her bottom is obscenely raised.

She lies for a moment, recalling that same position on Sunday. She is wet, and feels the nozzle firmly embedded in her behind.

She finds it quite natural to let her hand slide back down between her legs as she lies there, reflecting.

11. *If the Punishment Podium or Enema Chair are to be used, the recipient should position them in advance. In the case of the Enema Chair, she should ensure that the mechanism is working correctly, and that a graded series of punishment nozzles are available.*

12. *Similarly, if the occasion calls for the Sodomy Stool, the recipient should place the Stool in the spot reserved for it well in advance of her preparation for the ceremony in which it will be employed. When the Sodomy Stool is used, the recipient should also make the requisite preparations for the White Towel Test, and should ensure that the bedpan is available. The straps on the Stool, while not always required, should be tested by the recipient to see that they are in good working order. This is best accomplished by instructing her to bend over the stool and loosely secure the ankle, waist and wrist straps. A sodomy gown should, of course, be worn.*

"*Bête noire,*" she reads, "something one particularly dislikes or dreads." We all have them, snakes, bugs, political candidates of the opposite party. For all of us there are things that go bump in our night.

An often-overlooked truth of the *bête noire*: we can't live without it. Life without fears would be too safe, too contained. No great work of literature is complete without evil; good cannot exist without bad. For every white hat there must be a black hat out there somewhere waiting to ride into town after dark.

Lying on her bed, as she recalls what she has seen and heard, she realizes that she has felt both darkness as well as light. And that each has its appeal, or at least its necessity for the ceremony waiting to be performed.

The Sodomy Stool. The Punishment Podium. The Enema Chair. A sense of dread fills her as she mouths the words, afraid to utter them out loud. She doesn't know why, doesn't know if these things truly exist. She wonders at the alliterative power of the words.

Are they really just words?

Regardless, they are her *bêtes noires*, and she orgasms thinking about them. Fearing them and desiring them at the same time.

She shivers as she realizes that the reality of the situation is not far away.

OVER THE MILKING STOOL

We sat in a small restaurant not far from their house, discussing the problems they'd been having. Or rather that *she* had been having with *him*. They sat across from me, a pleasant enough couple in their early 30s, attractive, the woman talking, her husband sitting appropriately subdued besides her. He was a small man, in contrast to his rather tall wife; and he had that annoying habit of avoiding my eyes, especially when we came to the discussion of his malfeasance and its consequences, which were to be administered immediately after our conversation. Of course this is always the most difficult time for the culprit, male or female, the inevitable discussion of bad habits that precedes sentencing, and so I let him stare at his hands. There would be plenty of time for him to look me in the eyes later, when his wife had his underpants down for his medicine.

We'd talked already, more than once, so that we knew each other fairly well by the time we came to meet. I prefer it that way; intimacy is a prerequisite to chastisement: just as the student most fears a spanking from the teacher she or he knows best, my errant "pupils" obtain the maximum effect in a meeting with me after they've come to know me well, know what I'll tolerate and what I won't. And so the conversation was calm, with no surprises; and I drank my coffee as I took them in, observed how they interacted, noted the nuances of their behaviors, reference points that I intended to use later on that evening.

We talked about his behavior, and how his wife was tired of it. We'd been through it all before but it had a salutary effect on him to hear his crimes recapitulated. Mostly there was nothing fancy, sloppy habits and an inattention to household chores, all things resulting in more work for his wife. The kinds of things that you discuss with a fifteen-year-old. The kind of things that teenagers have been taken out behind the barn to "discuss" since before there were barns.

Mostly there was nothing fancy, but there were a few issues I could see were going to become the foci of correction. When I discipline — or supervise discipline — I believe there needs to be a rhythm set, with the biggest problems dealt with only after the smaller ones have been "discussed." A slow, inevitable progression, so that the miscreant always knows where he's been, and where he's going. I find that the anticipation is much greater that way. It's the best thing really: make him take down his underpants and listen to you and look directly into your eyes before you administer the strap; make him look at his red backside in the mirror before you stand him in the corner to listen while you run the water in the bathroom; make him stand there with his underpants down waiting, enduring a scolding while he hears you fill "his" enema bag, while he meditates on what he's got coming. And how the discipline he's about to endure is for something *serious*; and that all that, all the rest, while no laughing matter, was only a precursor to what's about to come.

So we sat and talked in that restaurant, his wife and I, while he sat there squirming on his seat, staring at his hands. He was, as I said, rather small, light complexioned, dirty blonde hair, slender. Long experience has made me a good judge of the bottoms of both sexes, a necessary skill for a disciplinarian. And I knew, without looking at his, that the evening's session would be rather severe. For slim he might be, but there was enough meat on his seat for him to take what he had coming. *All* of it. Which his wife clearly wanted to give him.

We talked, discussing his behavior, discussing their marriage, and when his wife had finished listing his crimes, I suggested we send him out to sit in their van and wait while we talked about what would be appropriate correction. I watched him hang his head as his wife spoke to him, "Billy," she said — his name was William, but I had suggested she use the diminutive form — "Billy, get up and go out to the van and sit and think about what the adults inside are discussing." He got up, and we both watched him go. I think his mind must have been on his bottom as much as his wife's was. We looked out through the plate glass windows of the restaurant as Billy opened the door of the family van and climbed inside. The door closed and Billy disappeared into the darkness of the interior. It occurred to me that he might be masturbating as he waited.

If that was the case, there would have to be additional punishment. I wondered if his wife had set up Billy's milking stool yet. The male version of the stool, the receptacle adjusted to Billy's proportions, the restraints attached and ready.

Well, there would be amply opportunity to find out.

❋   ❋   ❋

Billy, like most of the people I deal with, had been seeking discipline for as long as he could remember. And, like most of the people I deal with, his search had been largely unsuccessful, until he met me — or rather until his wife contacted me to ask if I would oversee a program of correction for him.

I don't say that with any arrogance; I am good at what I do, but I suspect there are others who may be equally as skilled. Quite simply, I understand the nature of discipline, why people like Billy seek it, and how it must be administered in order to satisfy their needs. I am an autodidact; but how can you be otherwise, when there is no training manual for what I do, when there is no one who has systematically examined the combination of psychology, algolagnia, inventiveness, physical presence and pure performance art required to give someone like Billy what he needs?

I can't give a single explanation of the need, some overarching theory that explains it. There are childhood factors of course: I've met and disciplined many people who grew up with strict parents and wanted to experience that same feeling of helplessness and comforting guidance as adults. And so I take great pains to inquire about that past. It's necessary, that understanding, letting the miscreant describe how he was sent to his room after dinner to wait, and how his mother came upstairs before bedtime to discuss his behavior with him. It's necessary, because having had these secrets revealed to me, I can exploit them — to his benefit — by recapitulating them. "Your mother sent you to your room," I might say to our hypothetical miscreant, and after he says yes, I will add, softly "I want you to do that for me now. Go there and think about what she saw when she came up, you bent over the back of a chair with your shorts and underpants down. When I come up — when your *wife* comes up, we'll expect to see the same thing."

And off our miscreant goes, with his mind already primed for what's coming, with those old memories and feelings floating in his head, welling up from deep inside him. It's cathartic, that reliving of old feelings as an adult, recapturing the positive aspects of discipline as parental love, while at the same time allowing for an adult consensuality.He's experiencing something more powerful than what he felt as a child, because he's submitting to it by choice. It's his call, to delve within himself, or to allow me to guide him to do so.

* * *

In the instant case, our Billy in the van, there was no sign of childhood correction. Our Billy was raised without corporal punishment, and his needs came from some other source, a strong mother I suspected, one that Billy loved as a child but never felt he had pleased. His wife and I discussed this in the restaurant, as we had discussed it before, but in the end I suggested that, whatever the root cause, it was clear that Billy badly wanted a more structured life than he had, wanted his wife to take a firm role in his behavior. Wanted to have her take his pants down when she thought it was necessary. And, happily, she wanted to do that for him. And for herself as well.

And so we discussed what needed to happen that night, how I was going to help her lay a groundwork for their disciplinary relationship that would give both of them what they wanted. For Billy. We talked about what forms reward and correction would take, and, after we had paid the bill, I took her out to my car and showed her what I had brought for her "discussion" with her husband. And I was proud of her for not blanching at what I showed her. After all, although much of it is for threat and nothing more — the gothic element, if you will — even so, most of it gets used.

We'll come presently to what got used that evening. I'm sure Billy was starting to wonder what he was in for when his wife got him out of his seat and had him follow us to my car to get the equipment out of the trunk and put it in their van. Not that it needed to be transferred; after all, I was following them home. But I had decided that it would be good for Billy to carry the bags, to feel their heaviness and to wonder what they contained. To keep his discipline in the center of his mind. Anticipation makes the drama more intense. The physical is not enough; if you want to take the culprit deep into his or her mind for maximum release, then you need to build that anticipation. Build the fear, build the tension. I never terrify the culprit; I direct his energies in a positive way. But even so the anxiety is there, anxiety, so that release, when it does come, is profound.

And that's what I was doing when I had him carry the bags back to their van and load them inside. That's what I was doing when I had him climb inside and sit there, listening while his wife scolded him with the door open, scolded him loudly as people walked by in the parking lot, shadows against the cold autumnal dusk.

That's what I was doing that evening, and that I had been doing with him almost from the beginning, when I had his wife set aside a room for his punishments. When I had her instruct him to furnish it with a juvenile bed and sheets and install several hooks into the bed itself and to the wall above it. When I had her make him note down each infraction in a "punishment book" that I knew he had carried with him to the restaurant.

I had been preparing him for this evening from almost our first conversation. And now, as I drove after them through the dusk, past rows of houses springing up out of the cold darkness, as I followed them up their driveway and parked and watch her get out and get him out of the back, as I watched him struggle under the load of baggage I had brought, I knew his tension was high.

Good, I thought. I've laid the groundwork. Under my supervision, his wife will do the rest.

I followed her up the path and into their house. She put the pot on to boil, invited me to sit down in the living room, and sent Billy upstairs to his room to get ready.

I watched him, hurrying up the stairs. I wondered if his wife also noticed how he clenched his buttocks under the thin fabric of the pants his wife had made him wear.

I heard noises from the upstairs. Downstairs, his wife made me a delicious cup of tea. I watched as she poured the hot water from the pot, watched the strong muscles tensing in her athletic arms.

I watched as she bent down to retrieve a napkin she had dropped, and imagined her bending over poor Billy as he lay waiting for her, kneeling partially naked over the milking stool. I imagined her pelvis moving rhythmically as she dealt with poor Billy over the stool, and then I took the cup of tea she offered me, and drank it, slowly and reflectively, as I listened to Billy getting ready upstairs.

I have found that there's nothing like a hot cup of tea on a cold evening.

❈   ❈   ❈

You won't find pictures of Billy's discipline anywhere, of course, but that's not to say it wasn't recorded. Oh no, quite the contrary. Discipline — the *ceremony* of discipline — needs to be documented, thoroughly. So that the culprit can be reminded of the penalties exacted upstairs in the little room when he misbehaves, so that the telling photographs can be put in the private album, kept in the dresser drawer and shown to him every night, to remind him of the rules that govern his behavior.

As a man, I feel I have some insight into the coarser sex. For a woman a photograph is both a reminder and a distraction. The women I have punished have always known in advance that their correction would be witnessed: by me; by an assistant if the procedures require that; by an audience if an instrument of correction as severe as the enema chair is required; and, in all cases, by the cold unblinking eye of the camera, of the videotape turning slowly as the chastisement proceeds. For a woman, that unblinking eye serves as a warning, a reminder that her punishment can be reviewed. That a later infraction might find her in her room on her bed in her punishment clothes watching the videotape of her previous discipline, seeing her behind turning red, seeing her own hands slowly reaching back to part her crimsoned cheeks for the nozzle — or often, for something larger.

But a woman will notice details that a man will not. She will blush at the sight of her behind, at her cheeks stretched apart, she will quiver at the thought of what happened. But she will also quiver if the view she presented was imperfect; and she will quiver if the label of her panties shows during her chastisement. And in that respect a camera is a distraction, so I use one liberally during correction, but when the culprit is a woman I am careful to ensure that she sees herself later only at her best. Not dry-eyed, mind you, not un-crimsoned. No. That would defeat the purpose of the camera, to provide a record, to imbed in the memory of the malfeasant the consequences of her crimes. But always, always attractive, always as an object to be desired, to be treasured, to be admired even in the most compromising of positions. And let me guarantee that my culprits are always in compromising positions when they are undergoing chastisement.

On the other hand, a man will see a photograph mainly as a reminder; he will look at his red bottom, he will see his hands parting his cheeks for the insertion of the nozzle; he will see himself standing in a corner with a rectal plug in what an Englishman would call his "bum" retaining; and he will be reminded of what he did, and what he got for it. And, if the photograph is being shown him as evidence of chastisements past, shown him as the prelude to chastisement present, he won't be worrying about the label he showed last time. No, dear friends, he'll be concerned about how the strap will feel across his bare cheeks, and how long he'll be made to retain the enema that he knows has been prepared — is being prepared — for him.

So let me assure you that Billy's chastisement was recorded, from start to finish, and although I have not released it for public view or comment, I have reviewed this recording carefully in preparation to writing. For to deviate from the facts would do a disservice to Billy, who received the punishment with relative dignity, to his wife, who administered it to him, and to you, the reader, to whom I owe a duty of full faith and candor.

Veritas.

Something I strive for.

* * *

The videotape opens with a scene of Billy's special room, his punishment room. As per my instructions his wife had set the camera up there, and as per *her* instructions Billy had turned it on when he was sent upstairs to prepare himself for correction.

The videotape opens with a scene of Billy's special room, and Billy standing mournfully in front of the camera, contemplating his fate. Such scenes are priceless, for they capture the internal dialog of the malfeasant, exposing the battle in his head over what is to come.

I've administered corporal punishment many times, and the process is surprisingly uniform. There is an equal mix of fear and desire; fear, because what's going to happen is painful and shameful; and desire, because the pain and shame bring catharsis. And so the culprit sits in the punishment room and waits, and as the culprit waits the fear and desire grow. The videocamera captures the nervous hands, plucking at the clothing, the special punishment clothes that lay bare the area bound for chastisement. And the look of anxiety in the face of the penitent, waiting to be punished and redeemed.

It's a very peculiar time, that interval alone in the punishment room, and it's unwise to truncate it without good cause. Better to give the penitent time to reflect, to experience the wash of emotions, than to short-change him or her by proceeding directly to discipline.

It's a peculiar time, and peculiar things happen during it. The chief one is arousal. You would think that the *last* thought in the culprit's mind would be sex, but I've seen too many damp patches or large bulges between the legs to have any doubt that such thoughts must often go through the mind of the condemned, as he or she sits there alone, listening to the clock ticking, looking at the belt in the closet, or the red rubber bag hanging down from the hook in the bathroom.

And such behavior cannot be allowed. Poor Billy in his room may not masturbate, because to do so would be to diminish the effect of the wait he is undergoing, to do so would diminish the correction he is about to receive. To do so would be to deny the absolute power of the chastiser over him, and that is not allowed. Cannot be allowed.

A masturbator caught should be punished. A compulsive onanist should be monitored closely, should be prevented from achieving self-gratification. I've put many a culprit to bed with her hands tied to prevent rubbing during the night. I've had many a naughty boy tucked in in coarse, itchy underpants, to discourage inappropriate actions. I've had to sentence many a culprit to a session on the milking stool before bedtime, something that is never a pleasure for me to do, or for the recipient, although of course the milking does cause pleasure as well as discomfort. I try to keep that in mind when I watch the culprit changing into punishment underpants, when I lead him or her to the milking stool and see the tears begin. I try to keep that in mind when I lock the culprit down over the stool, when I see the tensing of his or her pelvis during the final stages of the procedure, at the height of the milking.

I discourage onanism in a variety of ways. A videocamera in the punishment room before correction is the simplest, and it is certainly the most humane.

And it's important for a disciplinarian to be humane.

✳   ✳   ✳

By the time Billy's wife and I make our appearance on the videotape, Billy must have been alone in his room for about half an hour. During that time he had opened his closet door to reveal some of the instruments of correction his wife had placed there in preparation, and he had changed into his punishment clothes. ˙

Punishment is always a ceremony, and there should always be clothing reserved specifically for correction. My general rule is that the bottom should always be left bare by the clothing, but all the rest of the body should be covered; thus the culprit's mind is focused on his backside, and what's going to be done with it. Usually a hospital gown serves admirably for my purposes, but when I am dealing with a man it is often useful to require him to dress in more feminine attire, to emphasize the sudden change in status of his body, to make him aware of himself as an *object*, to force him into a more vulnerable self-conception.

And so when his wife and I walked into his room I was not surprised to find that Billy was now dressed as a woman, or at least in women's clothes, wearing a white shirt, skirt, and stockings. I knew without looking that underneath a garter-belt and punishment underpants completed the ensemble; and I also knew that, as per my instructions, Billy had been completely shaved from the waist down. He was smooth and shiny in the areas where it counted most.

Watching the tape now I see myself walking confidently into the room behind Billy's wife, staring for a moment at Billy, weepy already as he sits hunched over on the narrow little bed in his room, and then taking my own seat in a large comfortable armchair near the wall opposite Billy's punishment bed.

Punishment room. Punishment bed. Punishment book, punishment stool, punishment underpants, punishment gown. Punishment spankings and punishment enemas. Use these words with the culprit, and use them frequently. I do. The objects come to assume greater meaning when they are emphasized this way, when they are made part of a verbal ritual, as well as a physical one. And so I sat there in my armchair and looked at Billy, weepy already on his punishment bed in his punishment clothes, waiting for his punishment to begin.

And now I see Billy's wife walking towards her husband. She walks to the side of the bed and looks down at him. The camera doesn't capture the look on her face, but I know it's the look of anger and love. She walks to Billy, looks down at him and then nods to the covered tray on the little table by his bed. Billy blushes, and, like the good boy that he's trying too late to be, stands up without being told.

I see myself on the tape watching stoically, quietly, as Billy moves to the side of his bed while his wife places two large pillows near the edge. He lifts his skirt up at the rear. His punishment underpants are open in the back and, I know, in front, should a session on the milking stool be required. Slowly he bends forward over the side of his bed, and as he does so the flaps of his underpants part, exposing his behind to his wife and to me.

Slowly he bends, and as he does so his wife uncovers the tray by the bed and picks up a thermometer from it. Shakes it down. Opens a blue jar, and the room fills with the sudden strong smell of Vicks Vap-O-Rub.

She dips the thermometer in the Vicks as Billy, now prone over the pillows, looks up at her beseechingly. If I tighten my eyes I can almost imagine him as a young frightened girl, his derriere rounded by his positioning, his skirt seductively raised, his body shaved smooth. He looks at his wife with tears in his eyes. A pleading look.

Which she ignores as she calmly reaches down and holds his cheeks apart.

Neither she nor I comment as she pushes the rectal thermometer slowly and ceremoniously up her husband's bare bottom.

Billy, of course, whimpers as the cold glass rod slides in. The whimpering grows louder as he begins to respond to the Vicks.

Reviewing the tape now as I write, I see poor Billy squirming his behind from side to side to stop the burning he feels. I also see what I did not immediately notice then: a growing bulge in the front of his punishment underpants, a large lump that is quite evident when he shifts to face his bottom in my direction and I catch an unexpected view between his tensing legs.

I didn't notice his arousal. But his wife did, almost immediately. Poor Billy!

Because of course his bulge guaranteed a session for him over the milking stool.

Which on the tape I see quite clearly now, standing off to one side of the Billy's punishment room.

It's quite an ominous sight. Dark wood, heavy, brooding, the attaching straps unbuckled, waiting.

I designed it myself.

❊   ❊   ❊

Watching Billy squirm on the videotape, listening to his wife lecturing him about his behavior, it seems appropriate to offer up a momentary digression on the use of rectal thermometers.

I am a strong believer in the liberal use of rectal temps. And not just before discipline. Hardly. The beauty of a rectal thermometer, after all, is that it can be used in a diversity of situations, including but certainly not limited to disciplinary ones. And the mental effects of a good temperature taking can be made to include not just the fear that precedes correction, but also a sense of being loved, of being a child, and, if desired, of pure stimulation.

In preparation for our meeting, I told Billy's wife to get him in the habit of having his temperature taken this way. Of course when she did it she videotaped it, or took still photographs, so the documentation is before us. The young man on his tummy, the thermometer protruding lewdly from between his cheeks. Or the young man draped over his wife's lap with his underpants around his knees, her hand holding the thermometer in his backside for those long five minutes that he was told to remain still.

And in Billy's case — if Billy behaved himself during his temperature-takings — I told his wife that if he had been a good boy, if there were no demerits in his punishment book, then she could take him *in hand*, as it were. One hand on his stiffness, the other on the thermometer in his backside, rubbing, milking him gently as a reward for behaving. Again, so much different from a session on the milking stool.

Which, as I observed earlier, Billy was facing because of the problem he was having of keeping his mind on his disciplin,e instead of on the growing lump between his legs.

And I must note, viewing the videotape as I write, that that lump grows ever larger with each aggressive poke Billy's wife gives to the thermometer currently tickling him up his rear.

❋ ❋ ❋

Billy didn't move much as his wife withdrew the thermometer. Maybe he was too afraid; after all, he knew, more or less, what was coming, and that, combined with the shock of having this intimate act done before me and the strange sensation of being dressed as a woman, had to be affecting him.

I watch her on the videotape as she withdraws it, and I remember sitting in the chair watching her that night. This is always a turning point of sorts, as the thermometer is preparatory, even when coated with Vicks, while what follows is emphatically not.

Billy knew that too, because he had been told to take out the paddle and the strap, and he had sat on his bed looking at them as he waited for us to come upstairs. I'm sure he looked at them as well when he was having his temperature done, because his wife had thoughtfully placed them on the bed under his nose before she bent him over for the thermometer.

His wife withdrew the thermometer through the rear flap in his punishment underpants and held it up to the light. She read the temperature. Then, to his utter consternation, she also made a series of explicit comments on the cleanliness of the little glass rod that had so recently been in his backside.

I don't think I need to repeat exactly what was said — in fact it would be rather indiscreet of me to do so — but of course good personal hygiene is as important a part of a discipline regime as the washing up of dishes and the mopping of floors and all the other household chores that Billy had performed, negligently, if at all. And especially since Billy was there to have his bottom bared for correction, laziness in matters of the nether region was quite intolerable.

Which was the thrust of his wife's long lecture. Poor Billy. She stood him up for it, his skirt still pinned up in back, and I'm sure he tried his best to concentrate on what she was saying, but the Vicks that had coated thermometer was still having an effect in his backside. He shifted and tensed and clenched and cavorted, and I guess she thought he was mocking her, for about halfway through her lecture she suddenly drew her hand back and slapped him, smartly, across his face. Not enough to do damage, or really even to hurt, but the suddenness of it shocked him, humiliated him, and he burst into tears.

It is quite poignant to see a grown man cry like that. It doesn't happen without preparation — the kind of preparation Billy had undergone, deliberate, anxiety-producing. She slapped him and he burst into tears, and I was proud of how she handled it. She let him cry, because crying is cathartic and it's good for the culprit's soul to let some water out before the discipline proper.

She let him cry, but she *never distanced herself from him*. She stood near him, she maintained eye contact, she expressed disapproval, but in a voice that said "I know you're trying, but you have to try harder." She kept herself near him, let him feel her warmth as well as her disapproval. And that, in my experience, is the key to making the whole odyssey something more than a simple set of physical acts.

It's not just a spanking, you see, not just an enema. It's a mental thing, a feeling of being condemned, of being the object of anger, but anger with the prospect of redemption. "You've misbehaved, and you should be ashamed of yourself. As ashamed of yourself as I am of you." That's the first part, and the statement and the actions that accompany it should be tailored to the culprit. Should be carefully designed to penetrate his or her psyche, so that the full force of the message is received.

But there's the second part to the message, equally important, that the penitent *must* receive, and that's as follows: "I'm ashamed of you, and you should be ashamed of yourself. But you can do better.

You *can* and you *will*. And I'm going to help you. I'm going to punish you for what you've done, and you aren't going to want to sit for the next few days after our discussion is through. But after you've been punished you'll be forgiven. After you're punished we'll move forward with all of this and you'll do better. Because I'll have stiffened your resolve as well as disciplined your bare bottom."

That's the message Billy's wife sent to poor Billy when she slapped his face to get his attention, when she scolded him for not keeping his bottom clean for her. "This is not a joke," she seemed to say when she slapped him. "I care about you and I'm going to see you improve, even if I have to put you in girl's clothes and lift your skirt up and punish your behind every day for the next month." She actually said that. It's verbatim from the videotape.

And so she slowly and surely stripped Billy of his adult persona and took him back to childhood, to a childish state where he had no control apart from the control she allowed, where he was free to accept guilt and retribution without the layers of denial and illusions of self that cloak the adult. She took him back to childhood, to punish him. And he allowed her to, because he knew that, having been punished, having had the slate wiped clean, she would bring him back to adulthood, now cleansed of his guilt and shame. Punished, and ready to do better. Be better.

I was quite pleased with her. What I do is curative, pure and simple: the freeing up of tangled emotions, the overcoming of guilt, of inhibitions in a way that the mainstream doesn't understand, although they would perhaps profit from such cognition. And I was pleased that Billy's wife had learned the lessons I had taught her.

"Dominant, do no harm," I thought, repeating the old proviso to myself as I watched Billy's wife go to his closet and remove a tray. In the middle were two foil-wrapped lozenges. Billy was going to have his negligent hygienic habits attended to.

I wondered if I might slip back downstairs to refill that tea cup as I watched her unwrap the two suppositories on the tray and order Billy to bend back over the side of his punishment bed.

As he reached his hands back and spread his cheeks apart for her, as I watched the flaps of the punishment underpants part, as I observed her push the first glistening white bullet and then the second up his clenching backside, I decided against it.

She stood Billy up and marched him to the corner. The room was quiet. Billy was quiet too… at least at first. Then, as the suppositories began to work he began to shift from side to side. Like a child in distress, and for much the same reasons.

I call this the penitent's dance. But of course Billy was dancing a slow waltz in comparison to the jig he'd perform when she made him take the soapy bag enema.

I guess you'd have to add "dance instructor" to my long list of unlistable credentials.

✳ ✳ ✳

Now of course both Billy's wife and Billy himself knew that his punishments for the evening were going to include enemas. And, while Billy is shifting in the corner, feeling the growing pressure in his bowels brought about by the suppositories, it seems a good time to discuss the enemas he's about to get.

Yes, enemas. There should never be just one, because the ceremony of discipline should include both the application of the dreaded unknown and the equally feared corrections that have already been experienced.

Consider the cane, for example. The cane is severe, and it is rightly feared by a penitent who is about to receive it. If he has never been caned before, his dread will be based on what he's read about it, and about what he's imagined in his febrile fantasies. Seeing himself bent over, bare bum up and cheeks partially spread by the obligatory inward-pointing-of-toes that a caning requires. Everything between his legs is exposed; and his cheeks tense and dance as they feel the cold air on them. They clench and dance with each zephyr from the open window that he misinterprets as the descent of the cane.

He waits in fear of the first stroke, which is terrifying exactly because it is unknown. He waits and, when it finally comes through the air — the bowel-tensing *swoosh* that signals its descent — and lands across his bare cheeks in a throbbing glowing line of pain, the instrument is no longer just imagined. It's real.

And then, when the cane is raised again for the next stroke, the same tensing in his bowels, a tightening of his throat. For now he knows what to expect, and he therefore dreads it all the more. He knows what it's going to feel like across his bottom, he knows that the second red line will supplement the first. And, of course, he knows that the caning won't end with two strokes.

Thus, in a similar vein, there should always be more than one enema. To achieve the maximum effect the culprit should take one, which he will fear because he can only imagine what he will feel; and then he should be made to take at least one more, so that he can derive the maximum benefit from dreading that procedure before it is performed.

In the instant case, I had charted Billy's course through these untested waters (as it were) in advance with his wife, while Billy sat in disgrace and in anticipation of great discomfort in the family van in the restaurant parking lot. And we had decided that there would be a progression of invasiveness, ranging from rectal thermometer to suppositories, with a Fleet enema and then the bag to follow. As I've said before, anticipation is a major part of correction, and we wanted Billy to think long and hard about what was coming *before* it came. We wanted him to fear the thermometer before he felt it up his behind, and we wanted him thinking about what his wife would be filling in the bathroom before he saw her come out carrying the bulging red bag.

Taking Billy's temperature and putting him in the corner with two suppositories up his bowels was consequently a planned sequence of punishments, certainly not a haphazard one. From Billy's point of view a sequence had been established, one of incrementally more invasive procedures performed on his bottom. And this was our intention of course.... let the boy take his pants down in his room knowing he's going to be changing into his punishment clothes, let him take them down knowing there's going to be a thermometer tickling his bum hole, that there's going to be a thick glycerin suppository up there next, and a nozzle or two after that. It sets the right mood.

Moreover, it also prepares his bottom for whatever might need to be in store for it. An enema is easier to take after a suppository, since things are already… tidied up… by the effects of the suppository. And so at this point Billy is ripe and ready for the nozzle up his backside.

Except for one thing. I have a simple rule when it comes to enemas: the culprit's bottom *must always* be red before he or she spreads his or her cheeks for the tube.

Yes, it must always be red before the cheeks are parted for the insertion of the lubricated tube. Why? So that he or she derives the maximum benefit from the washout, and understands that it's punitive. Bad boys and girls get red bottoms before they get the tube. That's the rule. Also, from the point of view of the disciplinarian there's something very satisfying about seeing a red behind waiting for the nozzle. And so the disciplinarian should be certain that the culprit's bottom is red and stinging before the nozzle is put in.

"Bad boys and girls get red bottoms before they get the tube." Billy's wife said this to him, said it to the back of his head as he stood squirming in his corner. Said it slowly, and, after she was done, waited a long several seconds before adding, "Don't they?"

"Yes Ma'am," Billy replied, but his wife wasn't satisfied by his response. "What do bad boys and girls get?" she asked, sharply, and she drew back her hand and slapped his behind sharply before he could answer.

"They get red bottoms, Ma'am." Billy was practically hopping up and down at this point, so strong were the effects of the suppositories. His wife, confronted with the choice of letting him go to the potty or keeping him in the corner until he had performed to her satisfaction made the appropriate decision: she made him wait. I was quite proud of her.

"The *whole* sentence, Billy," his wife yelled, slapping his bottom again.

"Bad boys and girls get red bottoms before they get the tube," Billy stuttered out.

"And have *you* been a bad boy or girl?"

"Yes Ma'am. I've been a bad boy, Ma'am."

"Then what are you going to get, Billy?" his wife said, putting her left hand on his earlobe, her fingers forming a pincer on his soft yielding flesh.

"I'm going to get a red bottom… I'm going to get a red bottom before I get the tube. Ma'am."

"Good boy, " Billy's wife said, directing her husband out of the corner with a deft twist of her fingers on his throbbing earlobe. The inquisition over, she frog-marched Billy forward to his bed and pushed him down over the pillows, so that he was once again confronting the paddle and strap he had been told to take out of his closet and leave there.

Perhaps it would have been appropriate for Billy to receive a paddling then, while he was still feeling the full effects of the suppositories up his behind, but his wife took pity on him, and after keeping him there for a long moment — one that must have seemed like eternity to Billy — she let him up and let him go. And off he ran, barely closing the door to the bathroom behind him in his haste.

Of course it was the first and last time he'd be closing that particular door that evening.

❊   ❊   ❊

When Billy returned from the bathroom, shame-faced at our awareness of what he had done there, he came back to his small room to find his wife sitting on a large chair she had moved to the middle of the floor. Sitting on that chair, her arms crossed, the paddle and his punishment book on her lap. Billy returned to the room, dragged his feet across the carpet and came to a slow, hesitant stop in front of her, head down, red-faced with embarrassment.

As I watch him now, getting down on his knees in front of her, his face inches away from the book — which she holds open, letting him read each infraction aloud — I cannot help but see him as a penitent in the confessional, kneeling, repenting, waiting to atone, and to be forgiven.

Billy kneels before his wife, his face inches away from his book, reading his infractions aloud, looking nervously at the paddle. Billy kneels, reads, and squirms, for his bowels are emptied, but there are lingering effects to the suppositories that he is attempting to ignore. He kneels, he reads, and after he's read each crime aloud, his wife asks him if he knows what he deserves to help him remember to do his work, with diligence, without nagging.

"A spanking, Ma'am," Billy replies to each query. "A spanking, with the paddle you're holding. On my bare bottom." It's a ceremony, but there's no question that it's an effective one.

And, when the list of infractions has been recited, Billy is taken over his wife's lap, and finds himself gasping as her hand slips into the waistband of his underpants, her warm hand against his soon-to-be-warmed skin, caressing him briefly, and then stripping his underpants down.

I watch on the videotape as Billy lies, humbly, over his wife's knees, like a schoolboy over his mother's lap, bare-bottomed, in disgrace, waiting to be disgraced. His cheeks tense as his wife brushes her hand over them. She takes her time, lectures, scolds, her voice rising and falling, alternately filled with acid and with affection.

Another poignant moment, one that it's important to prolong, to ensure that the culprit is in the right state of mind when the paddle is raised in order to crimson his bottom. "This is for his own good." Repeat that to yourself, disciplinarian. "This is good for me." Repeat that to yourself, culprit. Both statements are true. And no amount of physical discomfort, no paddling, however lengthy, will achieve the desired release without that additional mental factor satisfied. So keep him there, keep her there, let the culprit feel the warmth of your thighs, the heat of your lap, the gentle caresses of your hand across the bared bottom, the pat of the palm as prelude to the hard whack of the paddle. Keep the culprit there, prostrate, head down and bottom up, until you are satisfied that he is in the right state to receive his medicine. Take his temperature again, make him reach back with his own hands to part his cheeks, have him stay that way as he tells you, in his own halting words, about the suppositories and how they made him feel. Keep him with his cheeks parted and scold him about what you see between them, and make him tell you about what he did in the bathroom after. Ask him if he understands that his privacy is a privilege not a right. A privilege that you intend to deprive him of, in order to make him a better boy.

And then spank him. If you feel he'll benefit from it, make him count each stroke. Apply the paddle slowly, unpredictably, allowing ample opportunity for scolding, for cajoling, for comforting. Alternate cheeks, predictably, and then in random fury. Be soft, be hard, be slow, be fast. Control him, let him squirm and then order him not to squirm. Spank him, not in anger, but in compassion, the compassion that comes from an understanding that this will truly help him. That he needs to feel you in control, that your job is to bend him to your will. Not for your own gratification, but for his own good. Spank him until he's compliant; if you know him well and know he'll feel your love as well as anger spank him long and hard until he asks you to stop. Continue. Until he begs you to stop, and you know that he's ready. Ready for the next step. For the Fleet. And the bag.

Billy's wife spanked him long and hard. Several times he turned his head towards me with tears in his eyes. I looked at his wife's face and saw love, and I saw her hand rise and fall mercilessly. Rising and falling, and Billy squirming and twisting as she spanked his bare bottom. His skirt up, his legs glinting from the stockings his wife had had him wear.

It was a chastened Billy who was sent to the corner after, who stood with his nose pressed against the wall, his bared red bottom on display, as his wife and I discussed whether a Fleet would precede the bag.

＊　＊　＊

As should be obvious, Billy's wife had given considerable thought to the evening's activities. Why? Because, for the two of them, Billy's need for structure underlay their interaction. With structure Billy prospered, without it he floundered. And their relationship rose and fell in synchrony with the structure in Billy's life.

How do you reach the conclusion you need this kind of externally imposed set of rules? There's no self-help magazine that advocates it, no easy conversation with friend or family that reveals it, no therapist (except perhaps the most broad-minded) who suggests it. So the simple answer is, you don't reach this sort of conclusion easily, if at all.

I've talked to many people who've felt the absence of something in their lives and, after perhaps decades of debate and denial, finally realized what they wanted. Maybe it's like being gay, knowing you're different in some way but without anyone to talk to who understands what that way is. Structure, control, externally imposed. It doesn't seem so complicated, does it? But of course it is.

We accept that children need structure; even the most liberal-minded parenting books are clear on this. And while punishment shouldn't be part of childhood, the same need not be said of the structure applied to an adult, to someone who seeks out a disciplinary relationship of his or her own free will. And yet, how do you come to realize that it's okay to want structure, to want discipline? How do you come to the point of feeling it's okay to want to be held responsible for your actions, to be rewarded for good behavior and punished for wrongdoing?

There's no easy answer to that question. Time, perhaps, and a growing desire that can't be quenched, will not be quelled. Time, desire, circumstances where you are allowed to escape the consequences of your actions, circumstances where, at most, you are scolded for what you've done, and find yourself wishing the scolding had turned into something else.

In this modern day such circumstances are increasingly rare. We live in a complex world and we're expected to exhibit "adult" behavior at all times. But given the stresses of modern life escape from that behavior has become even more precious now — even more necessary — than it was in the halcyon past, where a legion of strict parents, tutors, teachers, and friends waited to enforce rules and the consequences of errant behavior.

I don't look at myself as an anachronism, but perhaps in some sense I am. I am, after all, a firm believer in the peace that comes from old-fashioned penance, the kind that takes place in a bedroom, over a lap, or with the culprit bent shamefaced over the back of a chair as the disciplinarian's belt is unbuckled. And that is not a particularly modern view. But if I'm an anachronism, a throwback to the past, I find that I'm a *necessary* throwback, for my services are always in demand.

And Billy's wife and I had talked frequently about what I did, and I had found her a willing pupil, and a bright one. We had talked frequently before meeting, and now Billy was reading the rewards of our discourse.

In this case, the Fleet.

Which I see his wife holding in her hand now.

❊   ❊   ❊

Billy knelt on his bed with his head down for the Fleet. His head down and his bottom up in what in the medical profession is known as the "knee-chest" position. This position is useful when the fluid needs to go higher into the recipient's bottom; in Billy's case it was appropriate because of the exposure it subjected him to.

Not content with the humiliation Billy felt kneeling there with his bottom pressed back and his reddened cheeks spread, his wife had him turn his head to face us, and then, after studying the pathetic tearful face he presented to her, added that he ought to try to be a good boy. That he ought to try to be good by reaching his hands back to spread his cheeks while he waited. Which he did, his hands creeping slowly to his behind, pulling himself open for her, knowing that in doing so he was presenting the tight little target she would be probing with the nozzle of the Fleet.

Which, as I said, I saw his wife holding in her hand. A small plastic squeezebottle, with a flexible plastic nozzle screwed onto it. She stood above him, looking down at his bared bottom as she uncapped the nozzle. She had him watch as she slowly pulled the plastic cap off the nozzle, and she had him look at her as she scolded him about his behavior as she held the tip of the nozzle against the tight mouth to his bottom. She scolded him, and only when she had made him tell her he deserved to have the Fleet, deserved to have the nozzle pushed up his naughty backside, did she actually push it in.

What exactly is the sensation Billy experienced as the nozzle was inserted? This is one of the first questions I'm asked when I tell someone how I administer correction: "what does the nozzle feel like going in?"

The answer depends upon the size of the nozzle, and what's preceded it. A Fleet has a tip that's smooth and rather thin, so the sensation is like that of a thermometer, albeit a large one. On the other hand, an enema nozzle that can be found attached to a drugstore-style hot water bottle/douche/enema combination bag is larger still, both in diameter and length, and it's stiff, so the recipient will feel it more going in. And, when punishing a man, the length of the nozzle is especially significant because the longer it is the more it's likely to stimulate the prostate gland, which means the more likely it is to stimulate an erection. Much to the consternation of the recipient of the disciplinarian's ministrations.

Billy's wife was keenly aware of this fact, of course, and she pushed the nozzle of the Fleet deep into Billy's backside in order to maximize its intrusion up his bowels. She held it there a long moment and then began to squeeze the bottle. And as she squeezed the solution into his upturned, chastised, rump, she reached her free hand down between his legs, to where his masculinity dangled, and she gripped him tightly. Held and stroked him and he grew in her hand as she did, as he felt her stimulating him in front and tickling his prostate and his bottomhole in back. As he felt her forcing the contents of the Fleet into his red resistant rump.

I sat back and watched as he squirmed as she squeezed, as he shifted as she held the nozzle firmly in his backside and watched the fluid level drop. If I stop writing now and listen carefully to the sounds on the videotape, in the moments when Billy's whines and complaints trail off I can hear the sound of the fluid going in. For perhaps two minutes she squeezed, slowly, alternating pressure with pause to prolong his sensations of penetration. To let the slight pressure in his bowels expand, not to any intolerable level (that would come later), but even so a ratcheting up of pressure that would remind him where he was, and why he was there.

Finally she was done and the little plastic bottle was pressed almost flat. Admonishing her husband to be a good boy and retain, to hold it and not to move a muscle while he did so, she slowly withdrew the nozzle from his backside.

And Billy did indeed do his best not to move. No easy task, considering that his wife's hand had never left his tumescence, considering that she was stroking up and down his stiffness, carefully controlling his precarious balance between arousal and discomfort. Inviting him to approach orgasm, no, *compelling* it.

※　※　※

Now, a Fleet enema contains a chemical solution that causes a growing need to expel over the course of perhaps five to ten minutes, a sensation that grows stronger as time passes. And so Billy's wife rode him between the antipodes of stimulation and distress, stroking his penis as she let the pressure in his backside build.

Let's consider the scene precisely, let's build a word-picture to describe what I see now as the videotape plays. Billy kneels on the bed with his head down, his bare behind in the air. Feminine in his new attire he kneels, receiving his treatment. Feeling the discomfort in his backside, the soreness of his cheeks. His wife's hand stroking him as she scolds and controls, directing his attention to the sensations in his behind, to her hand and how it feels to be masturbated. How his punishment is deserved, is being recorded.

I can't count the number of times I've administered discipline to a patient in an artfully arranged hospital setting; arrived at some nondescript medical office building after hours, entered the elevator and ascended to the deserted suite of examining rooms and walked through an opened door only to be confronted by a scene much like the one I saw before me that night as Billy received his chastisement. The patient kneels, head down, bottom high, bared by the opening in the back of the gown or whatever clothing he's been required to wear. Through the open door the first sight of the bottom, up in the air, cheeks parted. The heavy sheen of Vaseline between them visible even from a distance. A filled enema bag dangling from an IV pole. A Fleet sitting, uncapped, in plain view of the culprit, waiting to be used. Perhaps the culprit kneels alone, or perhaps there is someone there to assist, a hand between the legs of the offender, a hand in motion, or a hand gently tickling, waiting for the command to be given to purge the offender of distracting sensations before the second — rectal — purge is administered.

I've talked to many nurses, and patient arousal is not uncommon during such hospital procedures; after all, the anus is richly innervated and, as I've discussed previously, both nozzle and fluid have a distinctly stimulatory effect in men and to a lesser extent in women. But of course in a punitive enema arousal is distressing, for it distracts from discipline. And thus for all the hospital-style punishments I've supervised or personally administered — and for Billy's correction too — arousal has to be dealt with before chastisement.

I could have arranged for Billy's wife to bring him to a clinic I knew of near their home, after hours, taking him out of the car and to the elevator dressed only in a hospital gown and slippers. I could have had her bring him up to the clinic and into the room that had been set aside for him, to have him kneel head-down on the exam table with his behind up for discipline, at her hands, or at those of a nurse.

I chose not to do that, though, preferring instead a home-discipline setting, letting Billy anticipate and fear a later trip to the clinic his wife might decide he needed. And so he knelt there in his punishment room, with his wife's hand between his legs, stimulating him as she noted his growing discomfort. Noted it out loud, commenting on it, adding that she could make him do it himself. Adding that, as we shall soon see, she was preparing him for his trip over the milking stool, and that he had to be nice and hard before he mounted the saddle of the stool for his ride.

For several minutes more she rubbed, letting him grow thick under her ministrations. Letting him grow as he groaned as he felt the pressure in his backside. Finally he had stiffened to her satisfaction. Still holding him firmly in her hand she instructed him to shuffle his knees back until he was off the bed. He complied. Still stiff, she marched him forward towards the stool. She had him stand by it, shuffling again from the pressure, the penitent about to be corrected for his lack of self-control.

She made him pull the stool out from against the wall, made him open the restraints, before she bent him over it, and inserted him into the receptacle in front.

He was still stiff as she bent him forward. I would have thought that fear would have made him limp.

Well, I've found that, even after all this time, there's always something new to look forward to in this line of work.

✻ ✻ ✻

The milking stool. It is, as I said, of my own design, crafted to gently support the restrained culprit in a position appropriate to the necessary task to be performed.

The ceremony of milking is one not to be taken lightly, although of course no aspect of discipline should be inflicted without thought behind it. In the case of Billy's milking, watching the tape now it seems best to transcribe the conversation and action it documents, to interpose as little of myself as possible between you, the reader, and the events of that evening.

Without further ado, then, Billy's milking.

✻ ✻ ✻

Interior, Billy's punishment room. Night time, and there are drafts of cold air blowing in from the closed windows, for it's that time of year. The narrator sits comfortably in his chair; across the room from him stand Billy, and his wife. Billy is wearing women's clothes, his skirt pinned up in back to reveal a blazing red bottom. In front his wife grips him tightly, squeezing on his stiffness to punctuate each point. The room itself is relatively bare, apart from a juvenile-sized bed against one wall, the narrator's armchair, a second, armless chair and, next to where Billy and his wife now stand, the milking stool. We fade in on the sounds of Billy pleading with his wife…

❋   ❋   ❋

Billy: Please… please. I *promise* I'll be good…

Wife: Please stop. I've heard that before. I've heard that one many times before, too many times to want to hear it again. You've earned this. It's that simple. And I want you to tell me that.

Billy: What?

Wife: That you've earned it. That you've earned yourself this entire discipline session. Say it now, Billy.

Billy: But…

Wife: *(Squeezing him hard in her hand.) Say* it. Isn't your bottom already sore enough to remind you about your behavior?

Billy: I'm… I'm sorry Ma'am… I *do* deserve this…

Wife: Why?

Billy: Why…

Wife: Yes, *why* do you deserve it? I don't want you to just parrot what I tell you, you know. I want to know *you* understand why you're here as well as I do. I want you to be responsible enough to take some responsibility for your actions.

Billy: Why… because… because I haven't been doing what I'm supposed to do. Because I don't take care of my responsibilities and I don't take care of myself and I don't take care of our relationship…

Wife: *(Loosening her grip and gently stroking. Billy hardens under her caress.)* No, you don't, Bill... and that's why you're Billy now. You know I'm doing this for your own good, don't you?

Billy: Yes...

Wife: *(Tightening her grip again.)* Don't you?

Billy: Yes Ma'am, you are.

Wife: *(Resumes stroking.)* Yes, Billy, I am. And you know I am... do you really want me to yell at you and to be angry at you and to make you feel guilty about it? Isn't it easier this way, isn't it easier having your pants down for it like a naughty child?

Billy: Yes...

Wife: Isn't it easier to be punished and then forgiven? And you DO want me to punish you, don't you Bill? You want to be Billy tonight don't you.

Billy: *(Hanging head.)* Yes. Yes... I do.

Wife: *(Stroking up and down, squeezing and then softening to emphasize each point.)* You *don't* want me to let you feel guilty. You *don't* want to be allowed to get away with things. You *don't* want to let this drag on. *Do you?*

Billy: No... *(thoughtful)*... No, I don't.

Wife: And we both understand what you need. We both understand what works for you, what form this needs to take up here in your little room where you're sent to be corrected. Don't we Billy?

Billy: Yes, Ma'am, we do.

Wife: It needs to take a particular form, of you, bare-bottomed, over my lap, or over the stool. Doesn't it.

Billy: Yes, Ma'am.

Wife: Where do you need to be?

Billy: Over your lap. Over your lap, or over the stool.

Wife: Bare-bottomed?

Billy: Yes.

Wife: *(Sharply.)* Say it.

Billy: Bare-bottomed. Bare-bottomed over your lap or over the stool.

Wife: Why?

Billy: Because I need it. Because I can't stand feeling guilty. Because I don't act the way I should sometimes, and when I don't act the way I should I need to be taken to task for that. I need to be taken to task, treated like a child, with limits set and enforced.

Wife: And is that for your own good, Billy?

Billy: *(Nods.)* Yes.

Wife: I do it because it helps you, don't I?

Billy: Yes, Ma'am.

Wife: And by helping you it helps us, doesn't it?

Billy: Yes.

Wife: *(Running her hand up and down his hardness, a loving caress that he quickly responds to.)* Tell me how.

Billy: How your being strict with me helps us? *(Closing eyes.)* I need this, it centers me. It's taken me years to realize it, to overcome the shame I've always felt about being different…

Wife: *(Gently.)* But you *aren't* different… you're just more honest about what you need than a lot of people…

Billy: Yes… maybe, but I don't know anyone else like me, don't have anyone to compare me to. All I know are all the people who just deal with all the problems they have like adults…

Wife: You *are* an adult, Billy. *(Puts free arm around him as she continues to move her hand on his shaft.)* How is it not adult to realize there are situations that you can't handle and to ask for help from me, your closest companion in dealing with them? How is that anything *but* adult? To have the strength and honesty to ask for that kind of help?

Billy: I don't know… if it is, then why don't other people do this too?

Wife: They *do*. You know that they do. We have someone here who's told us about others, people just like you, who need this just as much as you do.

Billy: I guess… I guess that's true.

Wife: Of course it is. *(Her voice becomes very soft, loving.)* It's time, isn't it Billy? Time for us to deal with your arousal. Time to get it out of your system.

Billy: *(Hanging head.)* Yes, Ma'am.
Wife: It's time for the stool, isn't it Billy.
Billy: Yes, Ma'am. It's time for the stool.
Wife: Come over here now and hold out your arms. Now
go down. That's my boy. Go down. Down. And over...

❄   ❄   ❄

And so she led him to the stool, and I watched as she bent him over it. Even in the subdued light the dark wood gleamed. She stepped back as he knelt down over it, put his hands forward, lowered himself down onto it. Slowly fitted himself to it, so that his hips were supported on the central pad of the saddle and his bared behind was raised up high into the cold air of the room as he waited for his ride. Even from where I sat I could see the goosepimples on his nether cheeks, partially from the cold, mostly from the fear he felt at what was coming.

He obediently put his hands forward, down to the front leg of the stool, so that she could fasten the restraints. A "stool" only in the sense that it has three legs, one at the front, with restraints attached to it for the culprit's hands; two at the rear, widely separated, with a restraint on each for one of the culprit's legs. As you can imagine, when fastened down, those legs are stretched wide apart, giving the chastiser easy access to the backside of the penitent, as well as to what's between his or her legs.

And Billy lies now, over the stool, and his wife steps to one side and flicks on a spotlight she's arranged earlier, the white beam of light cascading down, illuminating Billy's bared bottom, his white legs and red thighs and sore buttocks. The light illuminates his scourged flesh, the dark wood of the stool, the heavy leather restraints. It shines down on him, casts its light on Billy's behind as it waits to be purged.

Billy's wife reaches down underneath the stool, and unlatches the milking board. Holding it up before her helpless husband she applies Vaseline to the thick rubber donut in its middle, and squeezes the bulb that inflates the donut to make sure that it's working. She reattaches the board, and repeats the process with the rectal prong. Applying Vicks instead of Vaseline, of course, making sure the tube that runs down its center is free of obstructions, obstructions that might prevent the milking solution from being rapidly delivered to the recipient's bottom at the height of the procedure.

Having lubricated the prong, she attaches it to its support-arm and positions it so that its head rests just at the center of her husband's rear bullseye, teasing him there with the slight pressure that is a harbinger of its full intruding discomfort. She reaches under Billy and adjusts the milking board so that his stiffness is lightly gripped by the rubber donut, and steps back to survey her handiwork.

Their "conversation" resumes.

❊　❊　❊

Wife:　*(Looking down.)* You know what you have coming now, don't you Billy.

Billy:　*(Barely audible.)* Yes.

Wife:　*(Giving him a hard smack on his already red behind.)* I said, *Don't you, Billy?*

Billy:　*(Louder.)* Yes Ma'am!

Wife:　Much better. What are you about to get young man?

Billy:　A milking, Ma'am.

Wife:　Yes, a milking. Do you know what that is?

Billy:　Yes…

Wife:　It's to get your mind off your thing and onto your punishment isn't it Billy?

Billy:　*(Turning face so that it is no longer visible.)* Yes.

Wife:　Your thing. Your stiff thing. Your *penis*, Billy, your *dick*. What kept popping up earlier tonight, when your mind should have been on the disciplinary aspects of having your bottom bared for you. We're going to take care of that right now. Before you receive the rest of your correction. *(Resting her hand on his sore red bottom.)* So hot. So red. It's too bad you couldn't have behaved yourself earlier, so that I wouldn't have to do this now. After all you've already received… but I guess you need more, don't you, Billy?

Billy:　Yes…

Wife:　*(Pushing down on Billy's behind. Beneath him as he lies over the stool the head of his stiffness pushes forward slightly and into the Vaselined closeness of the rubber donut on the milking board. Billy groans.)* I said, you need more. Don't you Billy?

Billy: *(Groaning as more of him pushes into the tightness of the rubber ring.)* Yes... Ma'am.

Wife: Yes Ma'am. What are you saying you need more of Billy? Correction? Or that sensation you're feeling now as you push forward into that tight little hole?

Billy: *(Hesitatingly.)* I... I... correction, I was talking about correction...

Wife: *(Slapping his buttocks hard.) Were* you? I doubt that. Once again your mind's slipped from what we're here to discuss to other, wholly inappropriate matters. Your arousal isn't appropriate, Billy. But we'll be taking care of that soon enough.

Billy: *(Whimpers.)*

Wife: *(Watching Billy trying to thrust himself forward slightly without being noticed.)* You like that little hole, don't you Billy? Feels nice and tight, doesn't it. Well. You know how a milking works. You get to enjoy pushing your thing forward into that little hole in front while I get to enjoy pushing something forward into your little hole in back. (She gestures down to the rectal prong.) You get to tickle the rubber donut; I get to tickle your prostate.

Billy: *(Moans.)*

Wife: Only I don't enjoy this, Billy. I don't enjoy this because its not a reward for you, it's a punishment. And when you've been milked, I'm going to replace that prong with something else, that I'll have attached to me, and we'll continue this conversation, about your manners, and how they need to improve. And now let's see if we can't get down to the business of getting this further up your backside...

❊   ❊   ❊

At this point, Billy had managed to push himself further forward into the tight embrace of the rubber donut on the milking board. He would have pushed further, if only he had been able. But of course the design of the stool prevents the culprit from having such control. True, the position of the saddle relative to the milking board can be changed, so as to allow deeper penetration into the donut by the culprit — or, when its a woman over the milking stool, of the penetration of the rubber phallus on the milking stool into the malfeasant — but changes in the relationship of the board relative to the saddle can be made only by the person administering the punishment, not the person receiving it.

Billy was quickly aware of this fact, for strain as he might he could not lodge more than the first inch or so of his penis into the rubber ring on the milking board. He pushed forward, surreptitiously he thought, but both his wife and I saw his hips move and his buttocks tighten as he strained himself forward. *Smack,* his wife brought her hand down across his red raw rump, a sudden pain that brought with it an extra pressure down onto the ring that held him. A moment of pleasure, then the burn in his behind, and he relaxed, then tensed again to get himself more pleasure, earning himself another *smack*. Again the instant of heightened pleasure, again the swath of raw discomfort.

Now Billy's wife stepped back and picked up a heavy leather strap. The stakes were suddenly higher: every time Billy tried to move forward she brought the strap down across his behind. She was careful to swing it so that it landed above the point where the rectal prong teased his bottomhole; each time it descended it bit into his behind with a loud slapping noise and he flinched, thrust himself forward, feeling the momentary pleasure of the ring on him.

To add to the mix of sensations Billy was feeling, his wife now opened the jar of Vicks and, reaching down between his legs, applied a generous portion of the substance to the rubber ring in the milking board. And adjusted its distance from the saddle so that it was now closer by about three inches.

Billy's predicament was sudden, and difficult. The ring that had been so tantalizing for the pressure that it exerted was now anathama because of the coating of Vicks, but in order to avoid the ring, now so much closer, poor Billy had to push himself backward, away from it. And in pushing backward away from the ring he pushed himself forward onto the similarly lubricated rectal prong. Lifting himself up off the saddle by squeezing his legs, he avoided the ring, but the motion raised and separated his buttocks, and insured the penetration of the prong into his behind.

Billy's wife watched as Billy squirmed between the two unappetizing alternatives, alternately pushing forward onto the pressure and pain of the ring and then thrusting backward, sodomizing himself on the prong. And groaning whichever direction he took. For a long moment she surveyed her handiwork, and then stood up again and lifted the strap.

And then put it down.

And resumed the conversation with her husband.

❁   ❁   ❁

Wife: Now. I can't imagine you're feeling so comfortable, or eager to resist, are you Billy?

Billy: *(Groaning.)* Nnn... nooo...

Wife: I thought not. In fact, I think you'd be likely to agree with me that you'd like to be milked now, wouldn't you?

Billy: *(Groans.)*

Wife: Is that a yes? Next time I'll expect a real answer, young man, regardless of what's going on. For the moment though I'll take a grunt as a sign of assent. Correct?

Billy: *(Groans again.)*

Wife: Good. So then we're agreed that you need to be milked. Well, of course you know that with enough movement on that ring on the milking board you're going to have an orgasm, and since I had you sleep with your hands tied last night, and with no privacy privileges in the bathroom, I think we can safely say that there should be a nice present you have for me when that happens. Yes?

Billy: Yeee... sss...

Wife: Very good. I take it that means you haven't been touching yourself. I hope not, although I know in some young gentlemen and ladies the imminence of chastisement does lead to a compulsive need for self-gratification. But I know *you* are different. Aren't you? *(She pats his behind, pauses to adjust the rectal prong, repositioning it so that it is closer in to his bottomhole.)*

Billy: Yes...

Wife: Yes? Good boy. Now then. With enough movement on that ring you'll give me a nice present which we'll collect in the little container underneath the stool. In order to encourage you to perform, though, I think we'll give you what's often called a prostatic massage. Well, maybe not massage, but stimulation in any event... that's what the rectal prong is designed to do of course. Isn't it Billy?

Billy: Yes...

Wife: Yes. *(Suddenly sugary voice.)* You're doing *so* well, sweetheart. Let me just adjust this prong again. (She moves it closer in. Now there is no way Billy can avoid its penetration into his behind, and he lies face-down over the stool with an inch or so of the prong in his backside.) Now, where was I?

Billy: *(Groans.)*

Wife: You don't seem to be keeping up your end of our conversation, darling. Well, oh yes the rectal prong and prostatic stimulation. Well. Normally of course the bulk of the prong itself would be enough to, enough to shall we say *facilitate* your release? But in your case, I really think what would be even more effective is if you were to get a nice warm soapy punishment enema delivered through the prong during your ride, because I'm sure that the extra volume the enema gives and the nice tensing you'll have because of the soap will give you a very *thorough* release. Wouldn't you say that's so, Billy?

Billy: Pleaassseeee...

Wife: I'll take that as a yes. Very well then, I'll just go into the bathroom for a moment and get your bag ready. Don't go anywhere...

❋   ❋   ❋

Of course it was quite apparent that Billy wasn't going anywhere, trussed and tied as he was over the milking stool. So I sat quietly in my chair watching as Billy arched himself up and down over the stool. Down, to avoid the prong in his behind. Up, sodomizing himself on the prong, in order to avoid the clasping burning ring of rubber on the milking board. Up, down. Up, down he went. And as he did so I heard his wife turn on the faucets in the bathroom and run the water until it must have been warm. I heard her fill the bag, and I heard the familiar swishing sound of the soap being agitated in the water to get it to dissolve. Familiar, because I've done the same thing myself so many times. Stood in various bathrooms in various hotels and houses filling a multitude of enema bags with a variety of solutions that I'll soon be administering to a variety of naughty bottoms.

After a few minutes Billy's wife returned from the bathroom, holding the bag high as she walked. A standard red bag, what drugstores sell as a combination hot water bottle/douche/enema kit. The bag was bulging, and the white ribbed hose dangled down and swung as she walked back into the room. Billy, his head down, his mind on other things, didn't see her until she was at his side, and from his inverted position I suspect all he could see of what she carried was the ominously large open-end of the hose. But I saw how full the bag was, and, his wife told me later, so did Billy when she made him watch the tape after, in preparation for another discipline session she had to give him a week or so later. But that's a different story.

As I said, she returned from the bathroom carrying the bag, walked over to Billy and hung it from a hook in the wall that I hadn't noticed before. She slowly connected the hose to the end of the rectal prong and stepped back and bent down to address her husband, who by this time was fully cognizant of what was in store for him.

It should come as no surprise that, in the transcript I set out below of the conversation that followed, Billy's replies to his wife's questions were largely, if not utterly, incoherent.

* * *

Billy: *(Groaning.)*
Wife: Ah, I guess you see what I have in store for you. Shall I explain to you what's going to happen? No, don't bother to reply, I know you just want to hear what I have to say. So just keep your dirty mind on that pain in front, that discomfort in back. Now, as you know, this is the milking stool you're over, Billy, and you're going to stay over it until you've been milked. *Thoroughly* milked. Your behavior hasn't been good,

and you and I have both agreed you deserve to have your pants down for punishment, and tonight we're lucky enough to have our friend here *(gesturing to narrator)* to oversee your correction. And the unblinking eye of the videocamera *(gesturing to camera)* to record it. Clear so far?

Billy: Ungg…

Wife: Yes, I thought it would be. Very well then. You've had your temperature taken, you've been spanked, you've been given suppositories. And yet you're still aroused. I know its an uncontrollable response to some extent, Billy, but the *truth* is that you're here exactly *because* of your lack of control. So I'm not planning to go easy on you for your arousal, I see it as yet another manifestation of the same root problem of yours, no self-control. And don't bother to reply, because you know as well as I do that what I'm telling you is absolutely true.

Billy: Gnnng…

Wife: Yes. Now if you were a child and acted like this there might be some excuse for it, although I have to tell you that if you were a child and acted like this the honest truth is that you'd probably be punished, bare-bottomed, although not in the way you're being punished bare-bottomed now. But you're not a child, you're a grown man who *acts* like a child, not in all ways, but in enough to create a great deal of friction that doesn't need to be there, in enough ways to make my life more difficult, not to mention your own. And that's why you're here, Bill *(her voice becoming sad suddenly as she uses her husband's adult name)*, that's why you're here as Billy, with your pants down, dressed as a girl to make you feel humbled even apart from the humbling you should feel from the punishments.

Billy: *(Barely audible.)* I'm sorry…

Wife: What? You're sorry. Yes, I know you are, and you can consider this catharsis. A hard spanking, a good cleaning out, a milking, more punishment and then my forgiveness, all that guilt purged, a good cry and to bed and you will do your best to sin no more. Now, I'm not going to go on with this lecture, but I want to make sure of one thing before I proceed. And that's to know that you understand how much you deserve this. So you can tell me that now. That you deserve what you have coming. Take your mind off your prick and your ass long enough to tell me that, Billy.

Billy: *(Making an obvious effort to focus.)* I... yes, I... I do deserve this. Yes, I do deserve it. And I promise to be a better boy after...

Wife: *Thank* you. That's what I wanted to hear from you. Now, I've connected the rectal prong to this tube from the enema bag I've hung over you, because I want you to take an enema while you undergo your enforced masturbation, Billy. The volume in your behind is going to make you want to use the potty, my dear, but of course that's not going to be allowed until I say it's time. The enema is going to make you want to use the potty, especially because I've made it nice and soapy to stimulate a strong *urge* in your backside that you're going to find hard to control. But of course that's exactly my point, a physical demonstration of the need for self-control, the need for self-control that *you* seem to so lack. Understand?

Billy: Yes...

Wife: Now the interesting thing, sugarplum, is that as uncomfortable as you're going to be with that enema inside you, you're also going to be harder than you've ever been because of it. Chalk that up to pressure on your prostate. You're going to be hard and you're going to be aching to cum, and you will. When I let you. And when you do, it'll be the most thorough release you've ever had. But. But, once you do cum, once you're milked, that pressure in your bottom is going to make you ache for something else, for instant release, and that's where your self-control is going to be *very* important. That's when that naughty little mind of yours is going to get back to where it belongs, which is to focusing on your behavior, and your self-control and your ability to follow instructions. *My* instructions. Understand me, dear?

Billy: *(Groans.)*

Wife: Yes, that will do. Very well then, I'm going to start by increasing the pressure on your cock by inflating the rubber ring on the milking board just a trifle. *(She reaches down and gives the inflation bulb several squeezes.)* There, doesn't that feel nice? Well, apart from that Vicks, that is…

Billy: *(Louder groan.)*

Wife: Next I'm going to move the board a bit closer to the saddle so that it will be easier for you to ride deeper into it. Yes, yes I see you want to push your bottom backwards to keep from feeling that tight ring on you, to keep from feeling the Vicks. Don't worry, it won't do you any harm… but really, Billy, pushing back like that just makes you have the prong deeper in your red tushie. Is that something you like?

Billy: *No…*

Wife: No? I think you must be something of a bottom slut, dearie. Why, you seem to be doing your best to stretch your cheeks apart to get more of the rectal prong up your tight little backside, so I think you must really like that. Even with the Vicks on it, it feels so nice up there doesn't it? And every time you push back on it you feel it tickling your prostate, don't you? Every time you push back on it you get that extra throb in front from having that extra pressure in back. Don't you.

Billy: Yy… yyeeesssss…

Wife: *(Patting his bottom and then putting her hand on the clamp on the hose.)* Such an agreeable young man. My hand's on the clamp now, Billy, are you ready?

Billy: *(Groan.)*

Wife: Self-control. Let's have a complete sentence out of you now, or I'll give you the strap first! A *complete* sentence, my dear husband, but let me give the ring gripping your cock another good squeeze, and let me adjust the rectal prong so that its further up your naughty behind.

Billy: Please… oh *please*… yes, *yes,* I'm ready. Give it to me…

Wife: *(Hand toying with clamp.)* Give it to you? Give you your medicine?

Billy: Give me... give me my medicine, Ma'am... oh please, give it to me, shoot it into me, milk me...

Wife: Well, how *obedient* you are... I think I'll open this clamp and you can start your ride...

❋   ❋   ❋

The loud click of the clamp opening is quite audible in my ears as I review the videotape, although I remember that click quite distinctly without any such mechanical reminder, such were the events of the evening.

Billy tensed his whole body when his wife opened that clamp. I want to make that fact clear at the outset: that his whole body had been sensitized to this event, to its expectation, so much so that, when it finally came, the spasm passed throughout his whole body. And this is of course how it should be, how the whole evening had been planned, had been orchestrated. I've punished many people, not always with this degree of deliberation and forethought but, when circumstances allow for it, this is the best way.

Billy jumped when he heard that loud click, and he pressed himself tightly down onto the saddle of the milking stool as if he could avoid the inrush of soapy water by doing so. For a long moment he tenses there, pressing himself into the saddle, his cheeks tight behind him, trying to expel the hard rectal prong between them, to deny entrance to it, and to the soapy water that travels down its length and up into his entrails.

And then the discomfort of the ring gripping his cock set in. No doubt a momentary thrill, feeling that tight lubricated ring pass over his glans and then down the length of his shaft. Given the power balance between the two of them, Billy had never taken his wife's bottom, but the ring gripping him was as tight as any virginal bottomhole would be, male or female. No doubt his own rectum gripped the prong in it as tightly as the ring gripped Billy's cock.

Then discomfort set in, and he moaned and tried to raise himself up off the ring as the enema continued to flow down out of the emptying bag and into his chastised rump. He pushed back, up off the saddle, up off the milking board, and of course in doing so pushed his behind back onto the prong that impaled it. The camera angle doesn't adequately capture what his wife described seeing, doesn't adequately record what I myself have seen, more than a few times, when I have a culprit on the apparatus, and I watch the sudden lurch up, the cheeks forced apart by the unforgiving rubber in back, as I watch the length of the prong going up the resisting backside.

What did she see? She saw her husband, desperately see-sawing between the pleasure and pain of the rubber ring in front and the pleasure and pain of the rubber phallus up his rapidly-filling bum in back. Back and forth he went, up off the ring and into the phallus, down off the rectal prong and deep into the Vicks-coated ring.

You might say it's a second step in the penitent's dance I alluded to earlier, a second movement if you prefer. For a long while Billy thrust himself up and down, down and up as the bag emptied and the prong moved in and out in back as he moved out and in in front.

I should add, by the way, that I am quite pleased with the design of the milking stool.

Although I don't know if Billy would say the same…

* * *

Wife: (*Standing above her bucking husband, one hand on the clamp, staring up at the emptying enema bag.*) Well, you've gotten a good start on the bag, Billy. More than a start. It's almost three-quarters gone. And I bet you're nice and stiff in front with all that pressure in your backside… (*reaching hand down*)… yes, you certainly *are*. Well then, I think we're coming near to the point where you can't contain yourself any longer. But I have a warning for you: don't come without permission. Do you understand? If there's one thing I *won't* tolerate it's that, disobedience during correction. So you can buck yourself up and down as much as you'd like, and all the time you do that you can think about why you're having it, about listening to me and not that appendage between your legs. But *don't* come until I tell you to. If you do I'll punish you in a way that will make this look like a picnic.

Billy: (*Riding up and down, it is hard to tell just how carefully he is able to listen to what his wife is telling him.*

The bag is mostly empty now, and he is squirming and tensing as he tries his utmost to hold the water inside him.)

Wife: I'm going to start moving the rectal prong in and out of your behind now, Billy, as I talk to you. You can cooperate with me and push your bottom back for it, or you can push yourself down onto the saddle and away from it, but either way it'll go in, with our without your help. Turn your head now so that I can look at you as I do this. That's right. No no. Open your eyes and look into mine. Now I'm going to push it in very hard, and then I'll pull it out and push it back in. We'll get a rhythm going, like the rhythm of a farmhand milking a cow, squeezing its udder, massaging its teats, although I'm not squeezing you, am I. I could be I suppose, and if you're good through all this I might. Up and down, that's right. Lift your bottom to greet the rectal plug. *up* and *down*. Now you say, I've been a naughty boy, I have *been* a *naughty* boy, and I *deserve* to *have* my *ass* fucked by *you*. And each louder word, why I'll push the prong in nice and far in back as you say it. Start now.

Billy: I... have *been* a... *naughty* boy and I... *deserve* to *have* my *ass*... fucked by *you*...

Wife: Good. Let's check in front. Oh yes, very hard. Very close, Billy?

Billy: *(Nods head slightly.)*

Wife: Please *fuck* my *ass* and *teach* me to *behave*.

Billy: Please... *fuck* my... *ass* and *teach* me to... *behave*...

Wife: Closer. The bag's got about a quarter left. I'll leave it clamped until you're almost there... you can have an extra little encouragement to make you squirt... let's say your phrase again, Billy... Please *fuck* my *ass*...

✲   ✲   ✲

I think it's best if I describe what happened next, rather than continuing to transcribe the remainder of the conversation that Billy had with his wife. Why? Not because of any modesty on Billy's part, for what modesty he had at the beginning of the conversation had by this point long since passed.

No, it's just that a transcript could not do justice to what I witnessed in the final part of Billy's correction. The combination of sympathy and sangfroid that Billy's wife exhibited as she thrust the prong into and out of his bottom, in perfect rhythm with the sentence she had set him to reciting, "please, *fuck* my *ass* and *teach* me to *behave*..." over and over as she moved the prong in and out, brought him closer and closer to the brink he desired and feared for what would follow. I had taught her well, I thought, watching her raise and lower him on her voice, kind, then strict, lifting and lowering his mood, playing him towards the climax, as it were, up and down just as the prong moved up and down; just as *he* moved up and down on it and on the rubber donut that encircled him still.

And I was proud of Billy too, how he rode the stool towards that climax. How he did his best to cooperate, how he had abandoned himself to the sensations his wife controlled, and how he had abandoned himself to the emotional control she also now exerted as he rode.

And up and down he went, and in and out the prong went, and in and out *he* went through the donut, feeling its grip, feeling himself forced down into it and raised up out of it, and he came closer and closer to the brink until he was begging for release.

She denied him at first, and over and over again he repeated that sentence, "please, *fuck* my *ass*..." ringing through his punishment room. But he could control himself for only so long, and when that had come, when that time had passed, she told him to get ready. And told him to force himself down as hard as he could into the donut. And as he pushed into that tight rubber ring she forced the prong deep up his bottom, to the hilt. And as she did that, she opened the clamp.

And the remainder of the bag emptied into his behind as he screamed in his release, as he pumped himself into the rubber ring, as he was milked over the stool. He shuddered and shook and pumped and pumped and, when it was over, begged to be let up off the stool.

And this is the moment that was perhaps the most profound of the entire evening's ceremony. That moment when he begged for release after he had spent, when whatever fire of passion in his brain had been extinguished by his orgasm, when his world exploded and he came to feeling the pain in front, the prong in back, his sore cheeks and the volume of fluid in his backside.

He begged for release. And what do you think his wife did? Did she let him up and let him go? Or, did she continue his suffering, taking what was righteous retribution too far, turning strictness to cruelty?

Should I tell you? Or, like that famous short story, "The Lady or the Tiger?" should I leave it to you to decide for yourself?

Remember, in this business, the art of mystification is every bit as important as is the art of chastisement.

And you can add psychology, rhetoric, acting and, of course, skill as a scrivener to that list.

※　※　※

Well, call me a milksop, but here's what happened. Billy's wife lifted her skirt to reveal a harness, one she had apparently buckled herself into while she was in the bathroom preparing Billy's enema. She removed the rectal prong from its attachment, and secured it to the leather straps around her waist and legs. Reached under the milking stool and produced a pitcher of milky water I had not seen before. Poured the water into the now emptied enema bag, and as she placed the head of the prong against her husbands freshly violated bottomhole, I realized that the froth I saw at the top of the bag was there because the milky solution was soapy water.

More soapy water. More, since Billy already had a full bag's worth inside him.

Well. Call me old-fashioned, for I am a firm believer in intimacy between two loving adults. And so I got up and went downstairs to refill my cup of tea while the two of them concluded their conversation upstairs in that punishment room in that house in that Midwestern town on that autumn night.

The last vision I had of them was of Billy over the milking stool, with his wife pressing the stout bulk of the rectal prong back into his balky behind. Of the length of the shaft sliding up his backside, as he groaned and she talked to him, about her love and his capacity for good behavior.

And the last sound I heard, as I closed the door and walked down the carpeted passageway outside it and to the landing of the stairs, the last sound I heard?

The loud *click* as she opened the clamp on the hose.

AGEPLAY: FROM THE "PUNISHMENT BOOK"

A "Punishment Book" is, I've found, a very effective way of keeping track of a culprit's behavior and the penalties paid for misbehaviors of every sort. I once had a culprit I disciplined maintain such a Punishment Book; what follows is an excerpt.

❋   ❋   ❋

The doctor's office is a nondescript place, the sort of faceless building that you see everywhere, that as easily holds a branch post office or insurance agency as a group of doctors. Daddy turns the car into the parking lot, and I sit feeling my tummy tingling with discomfort.

I sit there watching as we slow down and Daddy brings the car to a halt, methodically putting it in park and turning off the ignition. I'm unhappy and uncomfortable for a number of reasons: because my stomach really hurts and has been for a while, the reason we are at the office, in fact; because I am very nervous about being there, because of what I think is going to happen; and, because Daddy is there with me, which makes everything ten times more embarrassing.

Before I have time to collect my thoughts, or to even have second thoughts, Daddy is getting out of the car and walking around to my side to open my door. It's a familiar motion, and usually it makes me feel calmer, feel like a little girl, but this time it doesn't feel that way. It feels like what it is, that he's coming to get me, to take me somewhere unpleasant, where something will happen that I don't like and don't want. But that I have no choice in getting.

I would say that it's the same feeling as when he comes to get me for a spanking, but I know that this is going to be worse. Much more embarrassing.

❋   ❋   ❋

Daddy opens the door and unbuckles the belt and takes my hand and helps me get up and out. I have to stand there in the mostly empty parking lot while he reaches in for the bag I've packed with my things, overnight things because the doctor has told Daddy that I may be there overnight for observations.

I stand there while Daddy gets my bag, feeling very embarrassed in my thin summer dress, feeling the hot air blowing on my bare legs and up underneath. There I stand, a young woman in an empty parking lot, with rows of blank windows in front of me, nameless horrors inside waiting for me.

❋ ❋ ❋

We go in through the front door, Daddy swinging it open for me and holding me by the wrist as he leads me in. It all makes me feel even more like a child, there with her Daddy for an examination of some sort. I fret as we wait at the front desk, looking around nervously at the mostly empty waiting room, a person or two scattered through the room, neat now in the early morning, magazines arranged, toys in the basket.

The receptionist finally puts down the phone and Daddy checks me in, speaking to her slowly, calmly, describing my symptoms to my chagrin, and I know my face turns red as he tells her what's been going on. I hang my head, and I am sure that the other people in the room can hear — are hearing — as he talks.

Daddy takes some time to talk to the receptionist, and when he's done he leads me to a chair to sit down. As we approach it I realize that it's where children normally sit: the toys are there and kid's magazines and books with bright colored covers and large attractive titles. Daddy sits me down and hands me one, "I Want My Daddy," which I dutifully thumb through as we sit and wait.

The book is more interesting than I thought, and I contemplate a career as a writer as I read it, perhaps writing for adults who like the simple structural form that children's books take. Simple words, simple harmonies, simple positive uplifting statements. The kind of gentle repetition that children delight in and that adults reproduce in their own absentminded rhythms. Without noticing it, I begin to rock slightly as I read, my lips moving as I form the words, "He came in a boat... He came in a plane... He came in a ship or a tug or a train."

❋ ❋ ❋

Daddy takes my wrist gently, and I stare down at his hand for a moment, and then realize that the nurse has called my name and that he is reminding me that it's time to come with him. Not a pleasant thought, and Daddy's hand — which would normally feel so reassuring — feels strange now. Foreign.

I get up and follow Daddy back to the front desk, where I stand while he rings the bell and waits calmly for the receptionist. She comes from the back holding a donut and a cup of coffee, which she sets down and disappears again, reappearing moments later to gesture to us from a doorway down the hall from where we stand.

Inside is a white corridor with carts at intervals along its length, and doorways on either side. I am led forward by Daddy, who is following the receptionist's lead, and in a minute I see a scale and a chair with a blood pressure cuff. A sphygmomanometer, I think, marveling at the complexity of the word, turning it over on my tongue as I absent-mindedly bend to remove my shoes and then step up on the scale to have my height and weight recorded.

Daddy, gentleman that he is, averts his eyes as my weight registers and the receptionist writes it down.

❋ ❋ ❋

The examining room is characteristically cold, and as we enter I realize that it is used for children. Fate... or is it cruel determination on Daddy's part?

And so I sit down on the examining table, which is absurdly small, although I am little enough to fit it, and I swing my legs the way a child does, looking around at the room, and the cabinets with swabs and tongue depressors, at the whales painted on the ceiling and the jar of lollipops at a side table.

❋ ❋ ❋

I sit and swing my legs and think about being a child, and let my mind wander back down the dusty lanes of memory. To a time when I was truly small and the world was much bigger than it is now, where adults were a separate tribe from us, gargantuans who ruled the earth and wandered through our world by our graces. Silently observed by us from our forts in the trees or our redoubts in the tall grasses that grew in vacant fields behind our houses.

Daddy takes my hand as I sit and I look at it, study it, marveling at the veins and the thickness of his fingers, and how small my hand is by comparison. On the wall is a picture of monkeys, and I look at my hand and Daddy's and then up at the picture and remember going to the zoo and seeing a newborn gorilla with its arms around its mother, who cradled it to her, to her bosom to let it suckle. Her tenderness human, or is it the other way round?

❋   ❋   ❋

The door opens while I am sitting absent-mindedly on the table, and in walk the doctor and his nurse. Daddy shakes hands, and they start talking about me, in a kind way, but totally ignoring my presence, which only accentuates my feeling of being little. Daddy describes the stomach pains I've been having, and tells the doctor that my diet hasn't been very good because of school. Pizza, macaroni and cheese, and other student fare.

I turn beet red and hang my head when Daddy goes on to tell his friend that I have also been very constipated, and that he's sure that's part of the reason for my stomach pains. The doctor tsk-tsks, and the nurse shakes her head from side to side slowly, and I wonder what she does when her kids suffer the same fate. I sit there, red-faced, waiting, while the adults talk about me, about my "problem" and how they are going to have to deal with it.

❋   ❋   ❋

Finally, it's time and the doctor walks over to me and looks into my ears and down my throat, and feels my glands while his nurse leaves the room to "get some supplies," she tells me in passing. So I sit, bravely holding my head still while the doctor pokes and prods at my head, with Daddy standing beside me holding my hand, rubbing it gently in his.

When the door opens a moment later, the nurse is there, pushing a small cart in front of her. Its contents are mostly covered by the white hospital gown she has draped on top, mostly, but not completely. And where it doesn't cover I can see enough to know what's coming, and I don't like what that is one little bit.

Underneath that gown, I see a latex rubber hose, and I know from experience that it's the hose of an enema bag. And as I sit there on the table, not swinging my legs now, terrified of the bag there under the gown, I hear, as if from a great distance, the voice of the nurse. Telling me, in what she thinks is a soothing tone, that it's time for me to come over to her so that she can put on the gown. I don't want to move, in fact I am frozen there on the table. But Daddy squeezes my hand in his and gently pulls me forward, lifting me up a little.

Against my will I move, sliding forward, standing, moving forward under Daddy's impetus towards the nurse who is picking up the gown and holding it out to me to step into. Undressed, of course. As Daddy undoes my shorts and I feel him slipping them down my legs, I stand there looking at the gown the nurse is holding out, seeing what's now completely exposed on the cart, how the bag is bulging and the water is opalescent with soap.

I am naked now and stepping forward towards the nurse and gown, and the doctor has picked up the bag and is hanging it, above the pediatric examining table. As I am walked towards it I see him picking up the Vaseline, and as the table comes nearer and nearer I wonder whether I will be on it, or bent over its end for the procedure. And then...

❋   ❋   ❋

... the scene shifts and I am imagining things from the point of view of Daddy or the doctor or his nurse. Or, as I imagine myself glancing around the room, from the point of view of an observer hidden in a supply closet looking through a peephole, like in a story Daddy once gave me to read. Through the limited field of view the young woman stands there, staring forward, her face red, looking at the nurse holding out the white gown, and the doctor off to one side, holding the open jar of Vaseline, methodically lubricating the nozzle.

❋   ❋   ❋

Slowly the girl moves forward into the enveloping whiteness of the gown, propelled forward by the gentle hand of older man standing near her, an intimate touch moving her forward like a rag-doll. The strong hand, first on her shoulder, and then, as she puts her arms out and the nurse begins to slip the gown on, the hand sliding down to the firm curve of her behind, a gentle, proprietary pat as the gown goes on and the nurse reaches around the embarrassed patient to tie it in back.

The girl moves forward towards the examining table, too small, and bends forward over its end, over a thick foam cushion that the nurse has placed there to get the height right. Bends forward, her behind high, the gown hanging open, her red face mostly hidden from view underneath her streaming hair.

❋ ❋ ❋

The room is cold, and there are goosepimples on her naked exposed bottom, and the harsh white lights of the room accentuate the contrast of flesh and white gown. Accentuate the gleam of the spotless counters and sink, of the metal bedpan, waiting, and of the IV stand with the heavy rubber bag hanging from it. Hanging down, tapering down to a long rubber tube ending in a thick nozzle the doctor is coating with Vaseline as the girl bends, helpless, over the end of the table.

Waiting.

For the inevitable.

❋ ❋ ❋

The view through the peephole is limited, but, by luck or by careful planning the girl appears centered of the narrow field of view, the doctor and nurse crossing in and out of view like lesser actors on a stage. Two characters in stage-center: the young woman, or rather her bottom; and the older man, standing to her side as she bends over the table, standing to her side holding her hand. Firmly, to prevent her rising. Lovingly, to give her comfort as she is held there to wait.

The doctor crosses into the field of view from the left and off again to the right, to the counter to one side of the table. His back remains in view, and his arm reaches up, and there is the sound of a cabinet being opened, the sound of a searching hand, and then the sound of a box being withdrawn and laid down on the metal of the counter.

The doctor mumbles something, and the nurse crosses over to help him, leaving the patient alone with the older man. A container is opened offstage, and there is the sudden *snap* of a rubber glove being stretched.

* * *

The doctor comes back into view, holding something in his hand, not visible because of the angle, but there is a flash, and then another as something metallic catches the lights from the ceiling. He approaches the girl's behind, and one hand reaches down to spread the gown further apart.

He says something to her in a soft voice, something inaudible through the little peephole, muffled by the acoustics of the room, and her bottom tenses. His hand comes into full view now, and in it is a hypodermic syringe, the plunger drawn back, a light violet liquid inside. The nurse comes into view, swabs a large portion of the girl's right cheek. The doctor raises the syringe, says something to the patient and plunges it in.

* * *

Her buttock tightens, accentuating the firm flesh, the doctor injects the contents of the syringe. When he is done he pulls the needle free, hands the hypodermic to the nurse and disappears back to the counter.

A moment later he returns to view with a fresh syringe in his hand. The nurse swabs the girl's other cheek, the doctor raises the syringe, the girl squeezes her buttocks tight and the doctor plunges the syringe in. He holds it there a long moment, waiting for the girl to relax her behind, and only when she has done so does he start the second injection. She lies there, over the cushion, face-down on the table, feeling the fluid being injected, unsure of herself, embarrassed, ashamed, squeezing her Daddy's hand like a little girl as the doctor prepares her for the treatment.

* * *

The second syringe is discarded, and the doctor disappears from view. When he returns he is holding a thermometer, shaking it down as he talks to the older man. The girl seems calmer now; her grip on the older man's hand is looser, and her rear cheeks are no longer tensed. In the center of each is a red spot, the entry point for the needle.

The nurse appears with the jar of Vaseline. The doctor dips the thermometer in and then holds it near the girl's head, speaking to her calmly and quietly as the nurse reaches out with both hands and parts the girl's cheeks.

The girl barely stirs when the thermometer goes in, feeling it as a slight tickling feeling, knowing how she looks there bent over the end of the table, over the cushion, her behind raised, her cheeks bare through the opening in the gown, the thermometer peeping out between them like a little flagpole.

And she lies there, helpless, three adults in the room with her. She is center-stage, and the doctor reenters the field of view. As the nurse looks at her watch, the doctor is reaching up to get the thick nozzle attached to the tube. He stands there looking at it, then dips it into the Vaseline jar. He moves to the girl's head, turns it gently and shows her the nozzle, explains its purpose.

He goes back to the end of the table, waits while the nurse withdraws the thermometer, reads it, and records the temperature on a chart. The nurse pulls the girl's cheeks apart and the doctor places the head of the nozzle against her small opening.

He begins to push it in...

＊　＊　＊

... and she feels it up against her, the gentle pushing of the pear-shaped head of the thick green nozzle. She tenses, unwilling, and the doctor feels her resistance, notes it, as does his nurse, as does the older man standing holding her hand during the procedure.

"The shots don't seem to be working," the doctor says, calmly, turning to his nurse as he speaks. "Lets try a direct, topical application of the medicine. I believe that the container is the one the second shelf of the controlled substance locker... you know the combination..."

He turns to the older man. "The easiest position is for her to be face-down over my lap. But, given her unease, it might be best if you're the one to do it... it's really quite straightforward, and I can show you..."

＊　＊　＊

The older man nods, and pats the girl's behind, two rounded cheeks bared between the two parted halves of the white gown. He helps her to stand, straightening her up as the doctor pulls a heavy wooden chair from a corner to the center of the examining room, the noise loud in the small room, masking the sound of the nurse fiddling with the combination lock on the metal cabinet bolted to the wall.

The doctor sits down on the chair, and gestures for the girl to come to him. She does, led by her Daddy, who watches calmly as she bends down over the doctor's knees, feeling the gown spread, feeling the cold air on her bare bottom, bending farther and farther until she is over his lap, bottom upwards, gown apart, waiting for the procedure.

❋　❋　❋

Or, rather, for the demonstration of the procedure at the hands of the doctor, the demonstration of the procedure that her Daddy will be performing while the doctor and his nurse watch...

And comment...

... and passing by in the corridor outside a nurse overhears those comments, and stops to listen, hearing the calm drone of the doctor explaining the purpose of the suppository, hearing the nurse coming back from the locked cabinet, her shoes making a soft clicking across the floor as she approaches the girl, approaches holding the waxy lozenge in her gloved hand.

❋　❋　❋

Perhaps the nurse in the corridor lingers a moment longer, hearing the soft calm voice of the older man commanding the girl over his lap to be still, to be brave; and she imagines the scene inside. The girl, who she saw briefly in the waiting room, face-down, gown open, cheeks pried apart by her companion. The doctor, a friend of hers who she can count on the recount the story later, or perhaps a lover who will tell her that night during their lovemaking, fueling her ardor with a recitation of the girl's embarrassment at the older man's hands.

The clock ticks on the wall, and with reluctance our observer resumes her rounds, hearing the sounds of childish complaints from the examining room as she walks away down the hall... walks away with her shoes *tap tap tapping* in time to the *tick tick tick* of the second hand of the clock...

* * *

... whose mechanical twin *tick tick tick*s along inside the room, marking the slow passage of time, time suspended or abnormally slowed, thinks the girl, hanging there, face-down and bared-bottom up over her Daddy's lap.

Time slowed, thinks the girl as her ordeal continues. *Tick... tick... tick...* as she feels his warm finger pushing in the waxy bulk of the suppository, holding it there a long, long moment. *Tick... tick... tick...* as she opens her mouth to wail, hears the sound leaving, in slow motion, like a train leaving a tunnel in a filmstrip played at quarter-speed, a favorite treat in grade school. *Tick... tick... tick...* and her world shrinks slowly, and she finds herself returning to childhood, keeping child-time: not one temporal stream but many...

... A fast-flowing torrent for the things she loves and wants, for ice cream and movies and sitting on Daddy's lap being read to...

... and...

... a slow, muddy, meandering Mississippi of reefs and sandbars and snags for things-to-be-avoided: report cards, the visits of wrinkled maiden aunts, meatloaf on Friday evening, cleverly disguised bible shows inadvertently found on a Saturday morning cartoon search and, most awful of all...

... a trip to the doctor...

... where she is now...

... lying there, feeling *it* in her bottom, feeling the pressure and slow dilation of her most intimate aperture. The sensation of it there, cool and unyielding, slowly dissolving. She lies there, face-down, studying the floor and the shoes of the doctor and his nurse, feeling the cold air blowing across her bottom, feeling her Daddy slowly smoothing her goosebumped peaches as she hangs there, feeling *it* dissolving inside her...

ABOUT THE AUTHOR

M.R. Strict is the pseudonym of a white-collar professional who has been an erotic enema practitioner and educator for several decades. Although his primary orientation his heterosexual, he has traveled worldwide to enjoy the practice of klismaphilia with enthusiasts of all genders and orientations. For further stories and ideas, visit his website at *www.intimateinvasions.com*.

BDSM/KINK

... But I Know What You Want: 25 Sex Tales for the Different
James Williams $13.95

The Compleat Spanker
Lady Green $12.95

Erotic Slavehood: A Miss Abernathy Omnibus
Christina Abernathy $15.95

Erotic Tickling
Michael Moran $13.95

Family Jewels: A Guide to Male Genital Play and Torment
Hardy Haberman $12.95

Flogging
Joseph W. Bean $12.95

The Human Pony: A Guide for Owners, Trainers and Admirers
Rebecca Wilcox $27.95

The Kinky Girl's Guide to Dating
Luna Grey $16.95

The (new and improved) Loving Dominant
John & Libby Warren $16.95

The Mistress Manual: A Good Girl's Guide to Female Dominance
Mistress Lorelei $16.95

The New Bottoming Book
The New Topping Book
Dossie Easton & Janet W. Hardy $14.95 ea.

Play Piercing
Deborah Addington $13.95

Radical Ecstasy: SM Journeys to Transcendence
Dossie Easton & Janet W. Hardy $16.95

The Seductive Art of Japanese Bondage
Midori, photographs by Craig Morey $27.95

The Sexually Dominant Woman: A Workbook for Nervous Beginners
Lady Green $11.95

SM 101: A Realistic Introduction
Jay Wiseman $24.95

21st Century Kinkycrafts
edited by Janet Hardy $19.95

GENERAL SEXUALITY

The Ethical Slut: A Guide to Infinite Sexual Possibilities
Dossie Easton & Catherine A. Liszt $16.95

Fantasy Made Flesh: The Essential Guide to Erotic Roleplay
Deborah Addington $13.95

A Hand in the Bush: The Fine Art of Vaginal Fisting
Deborah Addington $13.95

Paying For It: A Guide By Sex Workers for Their Customers
edited by Greta Christina $13.95

Phone Sex: Oral Skills and Aural Thrills
Miranda Austin $15.95

Sex Disasters... And How to Survive Them
C. Moser, Ph.D., M.D. & Janet W. Hardy $16.95

Tricks... To Please a Man
Tricks... To Please a Woman
both by Jay Wiseman $13.95 ea.

When Someone You Love Is Kinky
Dossie Easton & Catherine A. Liszt $15.95

TOYBAG GUIDES:

A Workshop In A Book   **$9.95 each**

Age Play, by Bridgett "Lee" Harrington

Canes and Caning, by Janet W. Hardy

Clips and Clamps, by Jack Rinella

Dungeon Emergencies & Supplies, by Jay Wiseman

Erotic Knifeplay, by Miranda Austin & Sam Atwood

Foot and Shoe Worship, by Midori

High-Tech Toys, by John Warren

Hot Wax and Temperature Play, by Spectrum

Medical Play, by Tempest

Greenery Press books are available from your favorite on-line or brick-and-mortar bookstore or erotic boutique, or direct from The Stockroom, www.stockroom.com, 1-800-755-TOYS.